T0329858

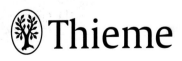

Osteosynthesis of the Hand

Instruments, Implants, and Techniques

Hartmut Foerstner, MD
Schramberg, Germany

In cooperation with Professor Ulrich Lanz

775 illustrations

Thieme
Stuttgart • New York • Delhi • Rio de Janeiro

Library of Congress Cataloging-in-Publication Data
is available from the publisher.

This book is an authorized translation of the 1st German edition published and copyrighted 2014 by Georg Thieme Verlag, Stuttgart. Title of the German edition: Osteosynthese der Hand. Bewährte Techniken für die Praxis

Translator: Geraldine O'Sullivan, Dublin, Ireland

Illustrator: Malgorzata and Piotr Gusta, Paris, France; Christiane and Dr. Michael von Solodkoff, Neckargemünd, Germany

With contributions by Professor Ulrich Lanz, Department of Hand Surgery, Perlach Hospital, Munich, Germany

© 2017 Georg Thieme Verlag KG

Thieme Publishers Stuttgart
Rüdigerstrasse 14, 70469 Stuttgart, Germany
+49 [0]711 8931 421, customerservice@thieme.de

Thieme Publishers New York
333 Seventh Avenue, New York, NY 10001, USA
+1-800-782-3488, customerservice@thieme.com

Thieme Publishers Delhi
A-12, Second Floor, Sector-2, Noida-201301
Uttar Pradesh, India
+91 120 45 566 00, customerservice@thieme.in

Thieme Publishers Rio, Thieme Publicações Ltda.
Edifício Rodolpho de Paoli, 25º andar
Av. Nilo Peçanha, 50 – Sala 2508
Rio de Janeiro 20020-906 Brasil
+55 21 3172 2297 / +55 21 3172 1896

Cover design: Thieme Publishing Group
Typesetting by Thomson Digital, India

Printed in India by Manipal Technologies Ltd, Manipal   5 4 3 2 1

ISBN 978-3-13-203811-0

Also available as an e-book:
eISBN 978-3-13-203821-9

Important note: Medicine is an ever-changing science undergoing continual development. Research and clinical experience are continually expanding our knowledge, in particular our knowledge of proper treatment and drug therapy. Insofar as this book mentions any dosage or application, readers may rest assured that the authors, editors, and publishers have made every effort to ensure that such references are in accordance with **the state of knowledge at the time of production of the book.**

Nevertheless, this does not involve, imply, or express any guarantee or responsibility on the part of the publishers in respect to any dosage instructions and forms of applications stated in the book. **Every user is requested to examine carefully** the manufacturers' leaflets accompanying each drug and to check, if necessary in consultation with a physician or specialist, whether the dosage schedules mentioned therein or the contraindications stated by the manufacturers differ from the statements made in the present book. Such examination is particularly important with drugs that are either rarely used or have been newly released on the market. Every dosage schedule or every form of application used is entirely at the user's own risk and responsibility. The authors and publishers request every user to report to the publishers any discrepancies or inaccuracies noticed. If errors in this work are found after publication, errata will be posted at www.thieme.com on the product description page.

Some of the product names, patents, and registered designs referred to in this book are in fact registered trademarks or proprietary names even though specific reference to this fact is not always made in the text. Therefore, the appearance of a name without designation as proprietary is not to be construed as a representation by the publisher that it is in the public domain.

To my teacher, Dr. Peter Reill

Hartmut Foerstner

Contents

Preface

Unimpaired hand function requires a stable bony framework. When fractures cause skeletal instability, this deficiency must be eliminated by targeted treatment, which may be surgical or nonoperative.

Every fracture must be assessed individually to determine the most suitable treatment. In each case, the benefits or disadvantages of surgical management must be carefully considered. Conservative management, where hand fractures do not need internal fixation, has often proved effective. Surgical treatment should only be considered when it is clearly superior to conservative methods.

The decision to perform surgery is determined by whether it will achieve the postoperative goal, namely, *early postoperative motion stability*. Only this allows the immediate initiation of hand motion, which, despite adequate surgical management, would be restricted by immobilization. If the goal of early motion stability cannot be achieved, the results of internal fixation are poorer than those of correctly-conducted conservative therapy.

Despite this warning, there are fractures that must be managed with internal fixation. These include:

- Fractures for which closed reduction is not possible
- Fractures which run the risk of redislocating, despite immobilization
- Open fractures with soft tissue injury
- Intra-articular fractures with nonreducible step-off
- Fractures that are unstable due to an articulation chain

The surgeon must sometimes accept a lesser degree of stability than early motion stability through adaptive osteosynthesis (Kirschner wire/adaptive screw fixation). Additional immobilization in the correct position is then required. Any restriction of function due to immobilization should be kept as small as possible or reversed by early, controlled therapy of the hand.

This book is based on 40 years' experience in hand surgery, with knowledge constantly updated during this period. Developments are critically observed and evaluated. The contents are intended to provide an illustrated overview of current internal fixation procedures in the hand. Methods no longer used today were also deliberately included as they may prove to be a saving alternative in a technical emergency. On the other hand, current methods that have often proved problematic because of undesirable side effects are also mentioned.

The lists of indications should facilitate the selection of a specific method for certain fracture types. They must not mislead the surgeon into regarding internal fixation as essential. The description of the individual steps may help to avoid technical difficulties during the operation.

The surgeon should respect the difficulties of internal fixation before embarking on an operation. Only through awareness of the pitfalls lurking behind internal fixation can these be avoided and the optimal benefits from surgical fracture management obtained.

Finally, conservative management carried out well is always better than poor internal fixation.

Hartmut Foerstner
Prof. Ulrich Lanz

Acknowledgments

Our thanks go to Georg Thieme Verlag for producing this work. A special mention goes to the project manager, Daria Wojciukiewicz, MD, for the excellent support and Antje Merz-Schönpflug, MD, responsible for editorial processing of the original German edition. Also thanks to Elke Plach for the technical processing and Anja Jahn who coordinated the artwork. For the realization of this English edition our special thanks go to the Editorial and Production Team, Angelika Findgott, Anne Lamparter, Jo Stead, and Martin Teichmann, and to the translator Geraldine O' Sullivan.

We are grateful to the employees of the Mediathek Schramberg, who managed to obtain originals of all the papers in the references, and the team at the practice of Dres Schoenemann, Gaus, Knöigsberger, Teufel, Fritz, and Fritz from Rottwel, for their great support. A very special thank you to Christiane von Solodkoff and Piotr Gusta, who produced the illustrations. They have all made a unique contribution towards the successful production of this book.

Hartmut Foerstner
Prof. Ulrich Lanz

Chapter 1

Introduction

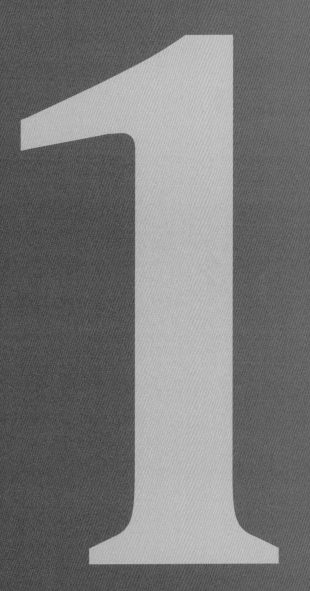

1 Introduction

1.1 General Remarks

▶ **Incidence.** Depending on the assessment method, hand fractures account for one fifth to one fourth of all fractures. The frequencies of fracture locations within the hand are classified very differently and factors specific for various countries appear to play a part in this. Fractures of the fingers and metacarpals are the most common, while fractures of the carpal bones are much rarer. Within the carpus, over 75% of fractures involve the scaphoid, followed by the triquetrum at just over 10%. Fractures of the trapezium, hamate, pisiform, lunate, and trapezoid each account for 3% or less.

The percentage of fractures of the hand in childhood is reported as up to 30%, which is a considerable number. Fractures occurring between the ages of 17 and 40 years occur predominantly in males. Nearly 50% of these occur at work and about 20% occur during sporting and leisure activities. This means that a very high proportion of fractures of the hand involve patients of working age. In this era of economic efficiency, the choice of treatment should ensure that workers can be reintegrated in the workforce as early as possible.

▶ **Restoration of function.** Considering the importance of the hand for daily life, the need for optimal management of hand and finger trauma becomes apparent. The aim is to achieve complete restoration of function by definitive treatment as soon as possible. All functionally important soft tissue structures (nerves, tendons, vessels, synovium, ligaments) must undergo primary surgical treatment at the same time whenever possible.

To restore function following fractures, the method (conservative or operative) that ensures the safest and fastest fracture consolidation should be employed so that functional rehabilitation is achieved as soon as possible. Among the available options, the treatment with the lowest complication rate must be chosen. This in turn demands many years of experience in hand surgery.

Since different operation methods lead to very different results with identical fracture types in different anatomical sites (finger ray and/or phalanx), the treatment that is most likely to be successful must always be selected for each location.

▶ **Early Motion Stability.** When surgical therapy is desirable, special attention is given to early motion stability.

Stability signifies the harmonious balance of complex static and dynamic systems. In the hand, these ensure the interaction of sensory and motor innervation, motor function, perfusion and static constancy, that is, the framework provided by the stable skeleton. If structural changes occur due to alterations of these complex harmonious systems, instability is produced where the original condition cannot be restored (e.g., loss of stability due to fracture). External influences and also disorders of internal dynamics can produce these structural changes.

Early motion stability, for instance when the skeleton is restored by surgical measures, is a state that still ensures the harmonious interplay of these complex systems even when affected by small changes and stresses. Before any decision on surgical fracture fixation is made, it is necessary to consider very thoroughly whether the goal of early motion stability can be achieved with the fixation.

Many fractures are sufficiently or relatively stable per se, for example, due to impaction, especially in the metaphyseal area, so that they are suitable for early functional management after brief conservative immobilization. These fractures should then be treated nonoperatively provided there is no significant axial deviation and/or rotation.

In such cases, closed and even open reduction often may lead to instability.

1.2 Recommendations

The following recommendations are based on a summary of empirical experience and experimental results in vitro and in vivo to provide rough guidelines:

▶ **Conservative treatment.** The most secure healing of a fracture takes place by secondary fracture healing (see Chapter 2.1). Prerequisites are fracture hematoma and adequate relative immobilization in the early phase along with sufficient stabilization in the transitional period between the soft-callus and hard-callus phases (see Chapter 2.1). Conservative therapy, applied correctly, meets these conditions. This means that *nonoperative treatment of fractures is the therapy of first choice.*

▶ **Surgical measures.** Surgical treatment may be indicated (see Chapter 4.3). However, the possibility that secondary fracture healing will be disturbed by an operation must be considered.

Thus, all percutaneous surgical procedures that do not interfere with the fracture and fracture hematoma are the next option. Percutaneous adaptive fixation (see Chapter 10.6, Chapter 10.10.3, Chapter 10.11, Chapter 10.13) and the external fixator (see Chapter 10.12) meet these requirements. The disadvantages of percutaneous surgical techniques include the need for additional external immobilization and, in the case of an external fixator, the complex care needed to avoid complications and possible lack of acceptance by the patient

▶ **Open reduction and internal fixation.** If surgery with internal fixation is absolutely indicated (Chapter 4.3), the following applies:

Joint fractures with a step-off must be stabilized without a step, if possible with inter-fragmentary compression (see Chapter 10.4, Chapter 10.6, Chapter 10.7.1).

Unstable metaphyseal fractures must be stabilized by internal fixation. Because of the relatively high healing potential of cancellous bone in the metaphyseal region, adaptive fixation usually suffices, as micromovements appear to promote fracture healing. An excessively rigid construction can obstruct healing. Fixed-angle locking fixation is permitted in the shaft region, if necessary at all, but is not absolutely necessary and is sometimes counterproductive particularly in the metaphyseal region.

Shaft fractures of long bones must be examined closely to see whether the fracture (transverse or oblique fracture) can be fixed by interfragmentary compression (see Chapter 10.7.1) by an appropriate surgical technique so that primary fracture healing can be ensured (see Chapter 2.2).

Additional neutralization of external forces is often required when a lag screw is used. It is achieved with a neutralization plate (see Chapter 10.5), which does not need to be a fixed-angle locking plate but can also be a regular standard plate or hybrid plate.

If fixed-angle locking treatment is considered exclusively, initially, interfragmentary compression of transverse and oblique fractures should be obtained surgically.

Whether the dynamic locking screw (DLS) or far-cortical locking technique will become widespread cannot be predicted at this time, especially in the area of the hand.

Extensive zones of comminution, especially in the tubular part of the shaft, require bridging internal fixation, although an external fixator (see Chapter 10.12) also can be considered. Bridging can be achieved both with a standard plate and with a fixed-angle locking plate. The latter may offer some additional advantages (see Chapter 10.7, Chapter 10.8).

There is currently consensus that plate internal fixation should be used with discretion in the *middle and proximal phalanges,* while it is used more in the metacarpals, along with intramedullary techniques (see Chapter 10.11).

Despite an optimal operation technique, there is a risk of postoperative limitation of motion, especially in the middle and proximal phalanges, due to scarring of the sliding layers of tendons and joints and because of the formation of callus, which restricts the use of internal fixation even if early motion stability can be achieved.

For *intra-articular dislocated comminuted fractures especially of the proximal interphalangeal joint,* treatment with functional extension/traction has proved effective (see Chapter 10.15), although early functional treatment produces astonishingly good results in the remodeling of the joint surfaces even in the case of nondislocated intra-articular fractures.

▶ **Conclusion.** If early motion stability is not achieved by internal fixation, nonsurgical treatment and possibly adaptive fixation are options with fewer associated risks.

Note

Internal fixation is indicated only if surgery can achieve early motion stability.

▶ Fig. 1.1 summarizes the treatment of hand trauma with fractures.

Note

The descriptions of internal fixation techniques in the following chapters should not mislead the reader into replacing nonoperative treatment by surgical fracture treatment. The different options for internal fixation will be described.

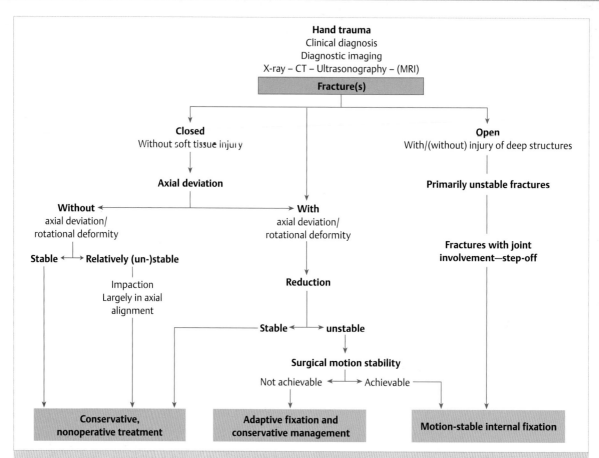

Fig. 1.1 Management of hand injuries associated with fractures. Algorithm for deciding between nonoperative treatment, adaptive fixation, or motion-stable fixation.

Chapter 2

Biology of Fracture Healing

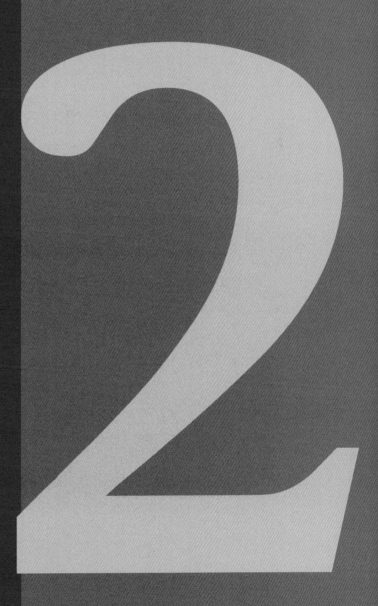

2 Biology of Fracture Healing

2.1 Secondary Indirect Fracture Healing

▶ **The healing process.** The natural course of fracture healing is secondary and indirect via the fracture hematoma to callus formation. This healing process takes place in four stages:
- Inflammatory phase
- Soft callus phase (approximately 2–3 weeks)
- Hard callus phase (3–4 months)
- Remodeling phase, consolidation (months–years)

The fracture gap is bridged by intramembranous and enchondral ossification in 3 to 4 months.

With fresh fractures, this healing process is started by the interplay of physiological, biochemical, immunological, and molecular biological factors. Besides the patient's age and sex, the fracture type (geometry and fracture gap), therapeutic immobilization (internal and/or external), and the subsequent loading influence fracture healing. Through dynamic osteogenesis, the bone mass, bone density, and bone structure adapt, under mechanical strain, to fit the situation. This means that dosed loading, adjusted to healing progress, must be exerted on the fracture during healing.

Mechanotransduction leads to the necessary molecular biological reaction, either through the macro- and microarchitecture (tensegrity theory) or alternatively proceeding from molecular and micromolecular structures to the macromolecular reaction (mechanosome theory). In each case, mechanotransfer leads to a molecular chemical reaction on loading, which is mediated through the three-dimensional network of the osteocytes. The healing process is thereby initiated (mechanocoupling, biochemical coupling, signal transduction from the sensor cells to the reactive cell, and its response—osteoblasts and osteoclasts) and regulated by cytokines, growth factors, hormones, and many other biochemical molecular substances. Mesenchymal cells from the bone marrow, along with induced angiogenesis, also play an important part in the healing process.

> **Note**
>
> *Relative stability* is a precondition for secondary fracture healing. This is achieved by external and/or internal immobilization.

▶ **Influencing factors.** Both fixation of the fracture and the type of loading can be influenced, but not the geometry of the fracture. This means that compression forces occur in a transverse fracture on axial loading and additional shear forces in an oblique fracture. Moreover, transverse forces, bending forces, and rotational forces can act on a fracture.

In mechanobiological terms, well-dosed interfragmentary movement in the early phase leads to faster fracture healing and hastens the transition from soft connective tissue callus to bridging, solidifying bony callus. In the later healing phase, however, tolerance to stress loading by interfragmentary movement diminishes considerably. Overloading then results in *hypertrophic pseudarthrosis*.

In comminuted fractures, stress movement is distributed to many fracture planes, so the individual movements diminish at cellular level. For this reason, stress movements are better tolerated in comminuted fractures (strain theory, Perren 2008).

In general, compression forces have a positive effect on fracture healing, especially if they occur in a cyclical manner. By contrast, shear, torsional, bending, and transverse forces delay healing.

A further important factor in healing is the size of the fracture gap. Even dosed distraction forces improve bridging of a fracture gap through the mechanism of intramembranous ossification.

Fractures in trabecular bone structures, such as carpal bones and juxta-articular metaphysial areas, heal mainly by enchondral ossification or combined with intramembranous ossification; bone healing is protracted. It must be distinguished from cortical fracture healing.

2.2 Primary Fracture Healing

> **Note**
>
> *Absolute stability*—stability also against major external stress—is necessary for primary fracture healing. However, absolute stability can only be achieved by internal fixation with *interfragmentary compression* and therefore almost exclusively in transverse and oblique fractures.

Contact healing of the fracture gap takes place through direct osteon growth across the fracture or healing of the gap through longitudinally aligned osteons that replace woven bone. No callus can be detected.

When a narrow fracture gap in a transverse or oblique fracture is overloaded by stress movements in the early phase, fracture healing reacts more sensitively: the result is then delayed fracture union or *atrophic pseudarthrosis*.

Fracture healing in the hand warrants several important comments:
- It is apparent in practice that no or relatively little callus can be detected by X-ray during healing of hand fractures.

- Secondary fracture healing appears to take place through a smaller fracture hematoma compared with fractures in other regions. Enchondral ossification to bridge the fracture gap tends to predominate. Therefore little or no callus is seen on X-ray. This also applies for carpal fractures.

The consequence is that phalangeal fractures can usually be regarded clinically as sufficiently stable with early motion after 3 weeks despite the radiographic absence of callus and still-visible fracture gap. Longer immobilization of these fractures is not usually indicated.

More prolonged enchondral ossification may be assumed in the wrist so immobilization for about 6 weeks is therefore indicated here.

The absence of tenderness in the fracture region is evidence that the fracture is largely healed.

Note

The absence on X-ray of callus in fractures of the hand, particularly phalangeal fractures, must not lead to excessively long immobilization.

Note

When fractures are treated nonoperatively, finger and wrist must be immobilized in the "intrinsic plus" position: 30% extension of the wrist, 70 to 90° flexion in the metacarpophalangeal joints, and a maximum of 20° flexion in the proximal interphalangeal joints.

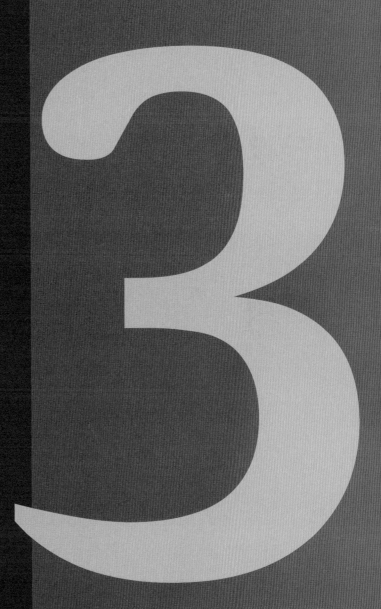

Chapter 3

Nonoperative Fracture Management

3 Nonoperative Fracture Management

Nonoperative (conservative) management of stable and relatively stable fractures in the hand remains important, especially for fractures of the phalanges. These continue to be treated by brief external splinting in functional intrinsic position combined with protected mobilization.

> **Note**
>
> The majority of finger and hand fractures can be appropriately managed with nonoperative treatment.

However, despite good bone healing, complications arise not infrequently due to the immobilization, which manifests as decreased range of motion, reduced strength, and residual pain. These require further special treatment to achieve the ultimate goal of a mobile, painless, functional hand.

Chapter 4

Surgical Fracture Management

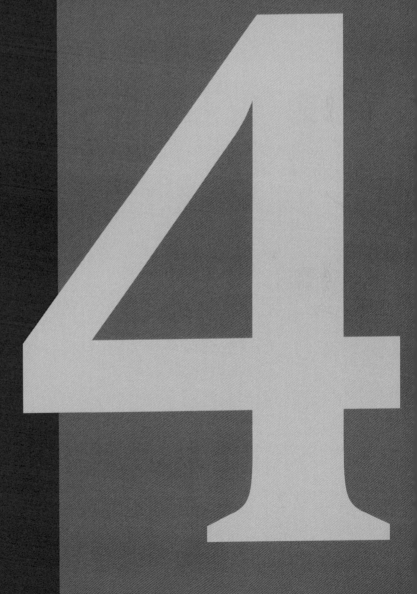

4 Surgical Fracture Management

4.1 Atraumatic Technique

Due to technical improvements in the materials used for internal fixation, the trend is toward surgical management of hand fractures (fingers and wrist), *provided that this confers an advantage in subsequent treatment.*

If surgical treatment of hand fractures is to have a better functional prognosis than nonoperative treatment, however, several important conditions must be met:

- A well-established operating team
- A surgeon experienced in hand surgery
- Instruments and implants of appropriate size
- Postoperative management by staff with specialist hand management skills

Note

Surgical management of a hand fracture is of benefit only if it achieves rigid fixation that allows early, active (protected) motion. In this case, functional postoperative physical therapy can begin immediately or a short time after the procedure. The goal is improvement of mobility, stability, and proprioception.

A further requirement is that adjacent structures in the hand that might be damaged by surgery are preserved by using *atraumatic operation technique.*

4.1.1 The Ten Commandments of Atraumatic Surgery

(after Nigst and Haussmann)

1. Thou shalt choose a functionally correct approach of adequate size.
2. Thou shalt know and identify the anatomy and proceed with dissection anatomically.
3. Thou shalt operate in a bloodless field using a tourniquet.
4. Thou shalt avoid all tissue distortion and therefore use sharp dissection and respect tissue planes.
5. Thou shalt not crush the tissue and thou shalt therefore use retaining sutures instead of retractors and sharp hooks instead of forceps.
6. Thou shalt use the finest possible instruments and sutures.
7. Thou shalt divide and crush blood vessels (including veins) as little as possible.
8. Thou shalt prevent tissue from drying out.
9. Thou shalt perform meticulous hemostasis (bipolar microthermy) and if in doubt apply a pressure dressing thyself.
10. Thou shalt make thyself as comfortable as possible at the operating table; do not hesitate to support thine arms and never look at the clock.

4.2 Common Injuries, Consequences of Trauma, Deformities

The more frequently occurring fractures can be explained by the type of force and by the anatomy. These largely determine the fracture type and deformity. An exact history of the accident and knowledge of anatomy are therefore highly important.

As mentioned in Chapter 1, fractures in adults often occur in the work setting. Fractures due to direct external force are usually combined with soft tissue injuries, thereby influencing the later functional result. For instance, this applies to saw injuries with open fractures, as seen in agriculture and forestry and among do-it-yourself enthusiasts and hobbyists. Shaft fractures, often comminuted, and intra-articular fractures result from blunt trauma.

4.2.1 Fractures of the Distal, Middle, and Proximal Phalanges

The typical fracture deformity in proximal extra-articular fractures of the *middle phalanx* can be explained by the anatomy. Owing to the pull of the superficial flexor tendon, the proximal fracture fragment is in flexed position while the distal middle phalanx fragment is pulled into extension by the extensor tendon apparatus with simultaneous flexion of the distal interphalangeal joint by the deep flexor tendon (▶ Fig. 4.1a).

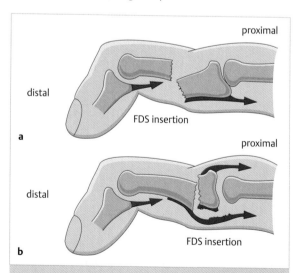

Fig. 4.1 Deformity due to proximal extra-articular fractures of the middle phalanx. FDS, flexor digitorum superficialis. **(a)** Fracture distal to the insertion of the superficial flexor tendon. **(b)** Fracture proximal to the insertion of the superficial flexor tendon.

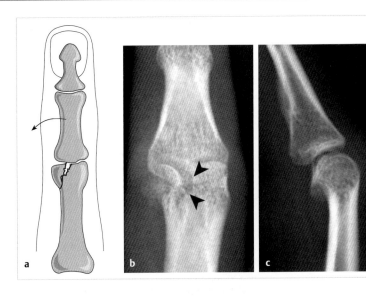

Fig. 4.2 Deformity due to distal monocondylar fracture of the proximal phalanx. Schematic **(a)** and X-ray in two planes **(b,c)**.

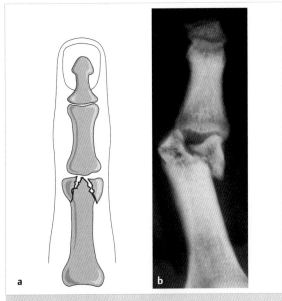

Fig. 4.3 Deformity due to distal bicondylar fracture of the proximal phalanx. Schematic **(a)** and X-ray **(b)**.

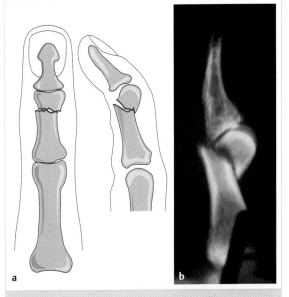

Fig. 4.4 Deformity due to subcapital phalangeal fracture in both planes. Schematic **(a)** and X-ray of subcapital fracture of the proximal phalanx of the thumb, lateral view **(b)**.

If the fracture is proximal to the insertion of the superficial flexor tendon, the distal fragment and distal interphalangeal joint are drawn into flexion by the deep flexor tendon (▶ Fig. 4.1b).

Closed and open injuries of the *distal phalanges,* sometimes with soft tissue loss or amputation, result from saw injuries and trapping of the distal phalanges by heavy objects.

Other types of fractures occur during sporting activities, especially ball sports. Axial stresses and lateral impacts cause intra-articular condylar fractures, basal fractures, marginal avulsions, fractures with tendon avulsion, and bony palmar plate avulsions.

Distal intra-articular fractures of the middle and proximal phalanges are often mono- or bicondylar fractures, which are associated with shortening and lateral deviation (▶ Fig. 4.2, ▶ Fig. 4.3).

Subcapital fractures of the phalanges tend to be hyperextended with lateral displacement (▶ Fig. 4.4).

Long *spiral fractures and torsional fractures* have a considerable tendency to shortening and there is often a rotational deformity (▶ Fig. 4.5).

With *proximal intra-articular fractures* of the distal, middle, and proximal phalanges, depressed and comminuted basal fractures must be distinguished from intra-articular

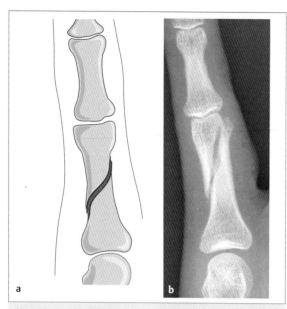

Fig. 4.5 Deformity due to long oblique fracture of the proximal phalanx. Schematic (a) and X-ray in one plane (b).

avulsions. Comminuted fractures of the base are characterized by shortening, a tendency to dislocation, radial/ulnar deviation and greater depression of the base on one side (▶ Fig. 4.6).

The size of the joint fragments plays an important part in *avulsion fractures*. The bigger the palmar/dorsal fragment, the more the tendency of the distal phalanges to dislocate because bony support can no longer be provided. The disturbed interplay between extensor and flexor tendon on the affected side increases the tendency to subluxation or dislocation (▶ Fig. 4.7, ▶ Fig. 4.8).

When managing these injuries, persistent impairment of movement of the affected joint must be anticipated, and it is essential to inform the patient of this possibility.

4.2.2 Metacarpal Fractures

Transverse and short oblique fractures in the metacarpal region tend to flexion deformity due to the tension of the flexor tendons (▶ Fig. 4.9, ▶ Fig. 4.10).

Subcapital fractures of the fifth metacarpal (boxer's fracture) are always tilted toward the palm (▶ Fig. 4.11). Because of the lack of palmar cortical support, this fracture tends to re-dislocate even after reduction. Unlike subcapital fractures of the second and third fingers, palmar angulation of up to 30° can be tolerated in the fifth finger provided there is no rotational deformity.

The abducted thumb and marginal little finger are particularly at risk in falls and because of axial impacts during ball sports. *Intra-articular fractures* of the base of the first metacarpal predominate (▶ Fig. 4.12, ▶ Fig. 4.13, ▶ Fig. 4.14).

These fractures dislocate because of the pull of the abductor muscles and/or there may be an intra-articular step-off. Since the muscle tension usually cannot be

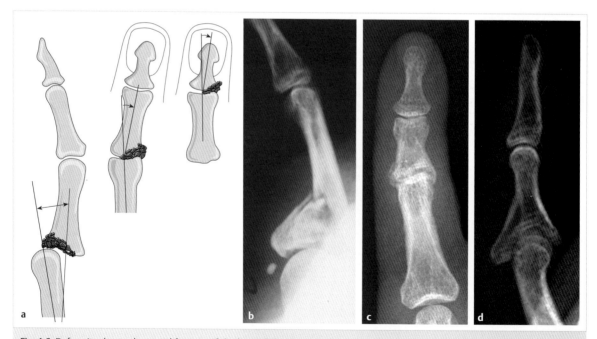

Fig. 4.6 Deformity due to depressed fracture of the base of the distal/middle/proximal phalanx. (a) Schematic. (b) Depressed fracture of the base of the proximal phalanx, lateral view. (c) Depressed fracture of the base of the middle phalanx, AP view. (d) Same patient as in (c), lateral view.

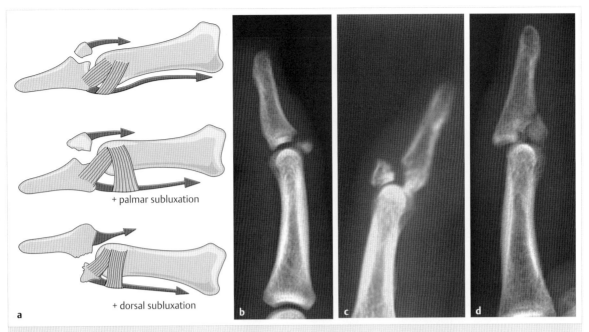

Fig. 4.7 Avulsion fracture of the distal phalanx. **(a)** Schematic. **(b)** Normal articulation with bony extensor tendon avulsion dorsally at the base of the distal phalanx. **(c)** Deformity with palmar subluxation due to a major dorsal avulsion fracture at the base of the distal phalanx. **(d)** Deformity with dorsal subluxation due to a major palmar avulsion fracture at the base of the distal phalanx.

(within schematic, image a)
+ palmar subluxation

+ dorsal subluxation

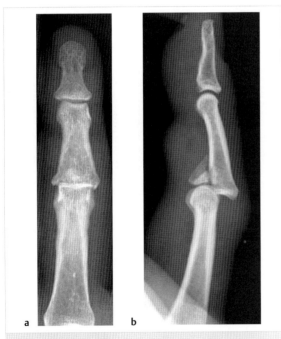

Fig. 4.8 Avulsion fracture of the middle phalanx, palmar.
(a) Major palmar avulsion at the base of the middle phalanx.
(b) The lateral view shows the dorsal dislocation of the middle phalanx.

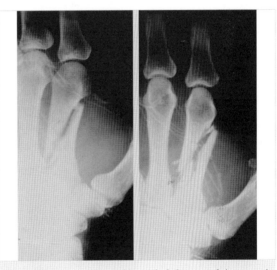

Fig. 4.9 Deformity due to oblique shaft fracture of the second metacarpal.

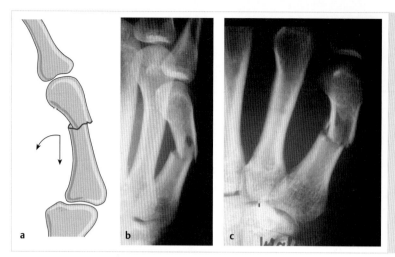

Fig. 4.10 Deformity due to transverse fracture of the shaft of the fifth metacarpal Schematic **(a)** and X-ray in two planes **(b,c)**.

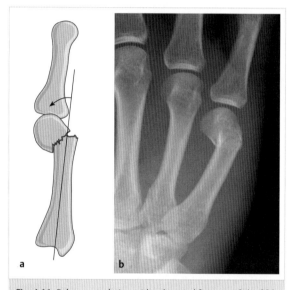

Fig. 4.11 Palmar angulation with subcapital fracture of the fifth metacarpal. Schematic **(a)** and X-ray **(b)**.

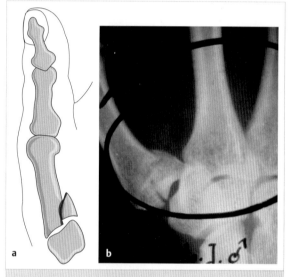

Fig. 4.12 Bennett fracture: palmar avulsion at the base of the first metacarpal. Schematic **(a)** and X-ray **(b)**.

neutralized by external immobilization, surgery is indicated. The same anatomical features of fractures at the base of the fifth metacarpal lead to an identical situation (▶ Fig. 4.15).

Skier's (gamekeeper's) thumb is a frequent injury. When the skier falls, the ulnar collateral ligament at the base of the proximal phalanx ruptures as a result of maximum radial abduction of the thumb (▶ Fig. 4.16). The ligament

is trapped over the adductor aponeurosis, giving rise to ligament instability that must be managed surgically. If the distal ulnar end of the collateral ligament is avulsed with a bony fragment of the base of the proximal phalanx, the ligament dislocation is obvious. Depending on the size of the bony fragment, stability can be attained by internal fixation.

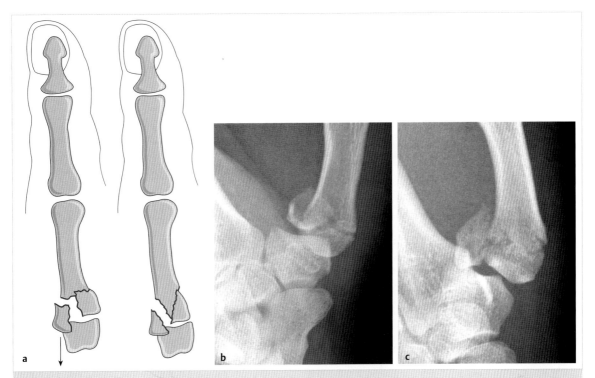

Fig. 4.13 Rolando fracture: intra-articular **T** and **Y** fracture of the base of the first metacarpal. Schematic **(a)** and X-ray in two planes **(b,c)**.

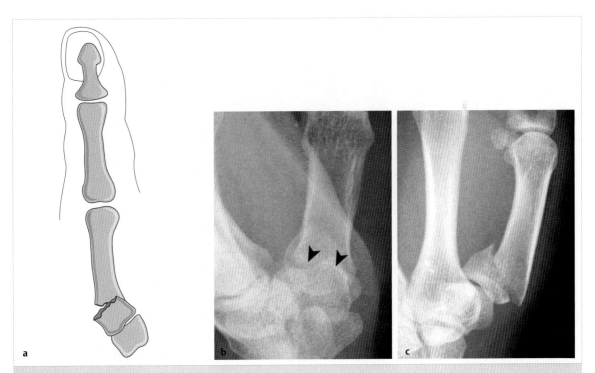

Fig. 4.14 Winterstein fracture: extra-articular transverse fracture of the base of the first metacarpal. Schematic **(a)** and X-ray in two planes **(b,c)**.

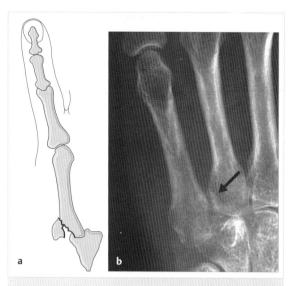

Fig. 4.15 Deformity due to intra-articular fracture of the base of the fifth metacarpal. Schematic **(a)** and X-ray **(b)**.

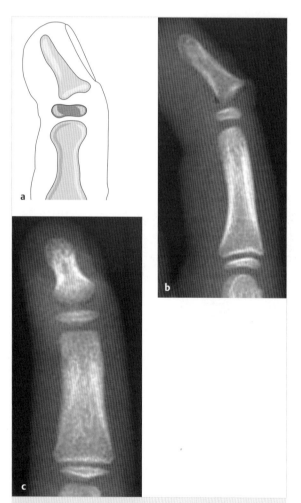

Fig. 4.17 Epiphyseal fracture in an 8-year-old child after a crush injury of the distal phalanx. Schematic **(a)** and X-ray in two planes **(b,c)**.

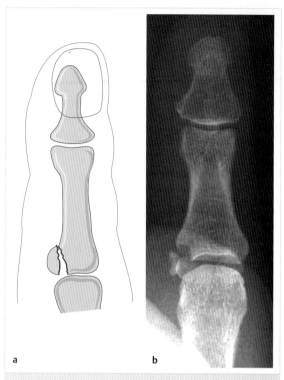

Fig. 4.16 Skier's (gamekeeper's) thumb. Dislocated bony avulsion of the ulnar collateral ligament at the first metacarpophalangeal joint. Schematic **(a)** and X-ray **(b)**.

4.2.3 Fractures in Children

A large percentage of fractures in childhood are the result of fingers getting caught. Bony injuries may be present even in the absence of skin and soft tissue injury.

Epiphyseal fracture dislocations at the base of the distal phalanx with dorsal displacement or angulation are typical (▶ Fig. 4.17). Clinical signs are subungual hematomas and fingertip swelling with local tenderness.

In *subcapital fractures of the middle phalanx,* which also occur after crush injuries in children, the distal fragment is pulled dorsally by the extensor tendon apparatus. This always results in considerable deformity (▶ Fig. 4.18).

Indirect *impacts* (falls from roller skates and bicycles) cause meta- or epiphyseal fracture of the *base of the proximal phalanx*. The little finger is affected in particular. The clinical sign is ulnar deviation, whereas the marked dorsal angulation is often hardly noticeable from the outside (▶ Fig. 4.19).

With these fractures, a degree of deformity in the form of dorsal angulation can be tolerated following reduction, provided there is no rotational deformity. Remodeling of the proximal phalanx due to growth is usually very good when the epiphyses are still sufficiently open. However, the parents must be informed about this.

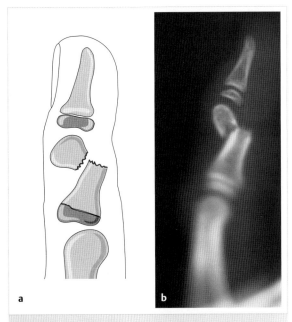

Fig. 4.18 Deformity due to subcapital fracture of the middle phalanx in childhood. Schematic (a) and X-ray (b).

4.2.4 Wrist Fractures

A fall onto the outstretched hand with wrist hyper-extended and high energy trauma (motorcycle accidents) are the commonest causes of wrist fractures. In the case of *scaphoid fractures* the clinical diagnosis is made from the tenderness in the anatomical snuffbox and the diagnosis is confirmed by special diagnostic imaging.

> **Note**
>
> Trans-scaphoid perilunate fracture dislocation must also be considered; surprisingly, this is often overlooked (▶ Fig. 4.20).

Fractures of the *other carpal bones* are rare but they are also often overlooked as their clinical features can be less obvious. They must always be considered in high energy injuries. Additional radiologic measures (CT, MRI) must be arranged.

Dorsal avulsion fracture of the triquetrum must be excluded with certainty after a fall onto the wrist if there is local tenderness over the dorsum of the triquetrum.

Continuous microtrauma of the hook of the hamate in racket sports (e.g., tennis) and golf can cause a fatigue fracture of its base. In this case, CT confirms the diagnosis.

The surgical indications and contraindications are presented in Chapter 1.2, Chapter 4.3, Chapter 4.4.

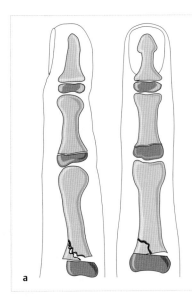
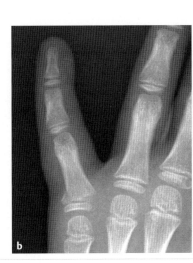

Fig. 4.19 Meta-/epiphyseal fracture of the proximal phalanx in a child. Schematic (a) and X-ray (b).

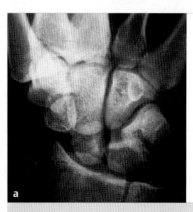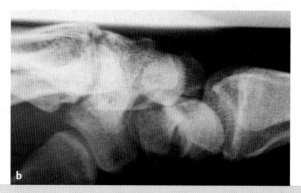

Fig. 4.20 Trans-scaphoid perilunate fracture dislocation. X-ray in two planes **(a,b)**.

4.3 Indication for Surgery

The following are indications for surgical management of bony injuries in the hand:
- Irreducible and/or unstable fractures
- Comminuted fractures
- Open fractures
- Fractures with joint involvement—step-off
- Fractures with irreducible rotational deformity
- Fractures combined with complex soft tissue injuries

If open fixation is indicated, the existing or anticipated iatrogenic soft tissue injury of other structures must be included in planning to allow for a potential changeover to external stabilization.

4.4 Contraindications

Contraindications to surgical management of bony injuries in the hand include:
- Insufficient bone substance and/or quality
- Florid infection
- Hypersensitivity to foreign bodies / metal
- Uncooperative patient, especially with regard to postoperative care
- Peripheral vascular disease, N.B. smoking
- Poor physical and/or mental health status

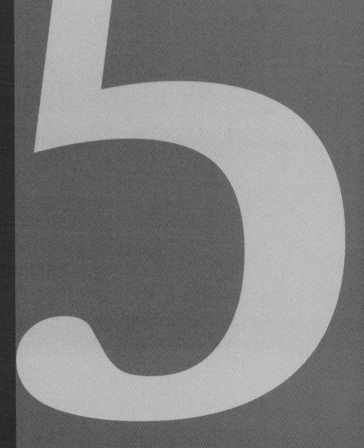

Chapter 5

Differential Indication

5 Differential Indication

5.1 Introduction

In this chapter, the most common fracture types in the hand and the current surgical treatment options are presented in tabular form. The first set of tables (▶ Table 5.1, ▶ Table 5.2, ▶ Table 5.3, ▶ Table 5.4) shows fractures of the distal phalanx, followed by fractures of the middle and proximal phalanges (▶ Table 5.5, ▶ Table 5.6, ▶ Table 5.7, ▶ Table 5.8, ▶ Table 5.9), of the metacarpals (▶ Table 5.10, ▶ Table 5.11, ▶ Table 5.12, ▶ Table 5.13, ▶ Table 5.14, ▶ Table 5.15), and of the proximal (▶ Table 5.16, ▶ Table 5.17, ▶ Table 5.18, ▶ Table 5.19) and distal (▶ Table 5.20, ▶ Table 5.21, ▶ Table 5.22) carpal bones.

▶ **AO code.** A brief explanation of the AO coding is as follows:

According to the general principles of the AO Foundation, fractures are coded according to their location and morphology. The first four numbers define the location, followed, after a hyphen, by a letter and number, which describe the fracture type.

- First number: 7 (identifies the hand as the location of the fracture)
- The second number identifies the **finger**:
  - Thumb 1
  - Index finger 2
  - Middle finger 3
  - Ring finger 4
  - Little finger 5
- The third number defines the **finger bone**:
  - Metacarpal 0
  - Proximal phalanx 1
  - Middle phalanx 2
  - Distal phalanx 3

In the **wrist**, the second number codes the proximal (6) and distal (7) row and the third number identifies the individual carpal bones from radial to ulnar:

- Scaphoid 61
- Lunate 62
- Triquetrum 63
- Pisiform 64
- Trapezium 71
- Trapezoid 72
- Capitate 73
- Hamate 74
- The fourth number, separated by a period, identifies the location **within the bone:**
  - Proximal 1
  - Diaphyseal, shaft 2
  - Distal 3

A letter and a further number, separated from the first three numbers by a hyphen, describes the **fracture type:**

- Carpus:
  - A1: avulsion, A2: chip, A3: comminuted
  - With reference to the forearm axis: B1: transverse, B2: spiral, B3: parallel
  - With regard to the number of fragments: C1: with a third fragment, C2: multiple fragments, C3: comminuted
- Metacarpal, proximal phalanx, middle phalanx, distal phalanx:
  - A = diaphyseal: 1 simple, 2: with a third fragment, 3: multifragmentary
  - B = metaphyseal: 1 simple, 2: with a third fragment, 3: multifragmentary
  - C = intra-articular fracture: 1: unicondylar, 2: bicondylar, 3: multifragmentary, depression

Additional Information

The author would like to emphasize that the listed operation methods represent a treatment possibility *only* if **surgery is indicated**. The limiting factors are defined in Chapter 4.3 and Chapter 4.4.

Moreover, ▶ Fig. 1.1 shows an algorithm for deciding on therapy.

The radiographs show only the variety of fracture geometries and fracture types. Each must be considered individually to establish which of the possible treatment options may be appropriate.

5.2 Distal Phalanx Fractures

5.2.1 Fractures of the Distal Phalanx, Distal

Table 5.1 Distal phalanx fractures, distal

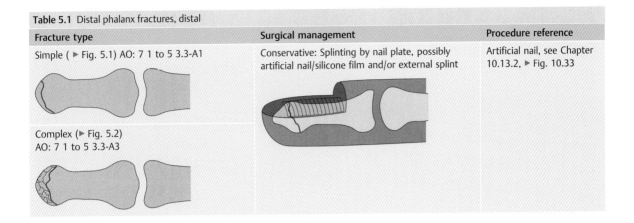

Fracture type	Surgical management	Procedure reference
Simple (▶ Fig. 5.1) AO: 7 1 to 5 3.3-A1	Conservative: Splinting by nail plate, possibly artificial nail/silicone film and/or external splint	Artificial nail, see Chapter 10.13.2, ▶ Fig. 10.33
Complex (▶ Fig. 5.2) AO: 7 1 to 5 3.3-A3		

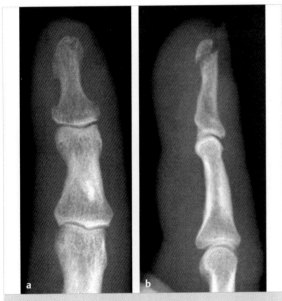

Fig. 5.1 Distal phalanx fracture, distal, simple. Right fifth finger, X-ray in two planes (a,b).

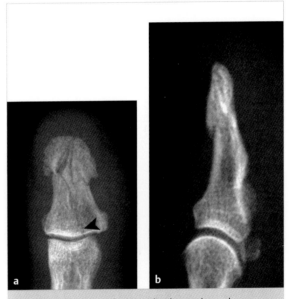

Fig. 5.2 Distal phalanx fracture, distal, complex and intra-articular longitudinal fracture. Right thumb, X-ray in two planes (a,b).

5.2.2 Fractures of the Distal Phalanx Shaft

Table 5.2 Distal phalanx shaft fractures

Fracture type	Surgical management	Procedure reference
Simple transverse (▶ Fig. 5.3) AO: 7 1 to 5 3.2-A1	Conservative: Splinting by nail plate, possibly artificial nail and/or external splint	
Simple spiral, longitudinal (▶ Fig. 5.4) AO: 7 1 to 5 3.2-A1/A2		
Complex (▶ Fig. 5.5) AO: 7 1 to 5 3.2-A3	Percutaneous Kirschner wire occasionally	See Chapter 10.13.2

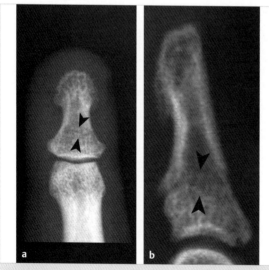

Fig. 5.3 Distal phalanx shaft fracture, transverse. Right fifth finger, X-ray in two planes (a,b).

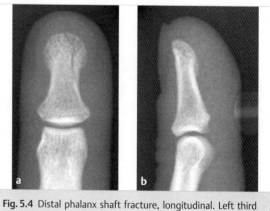

Fig. 5.4 Distal phalanx shaft fracture, longitudinal. Left third finger, X-ray in two planes (a,b), see also Fig. 5.2.

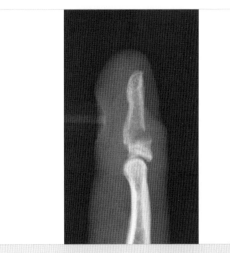

Fig. 5.6 Extra-articular distal phalanx fracture, proximal.

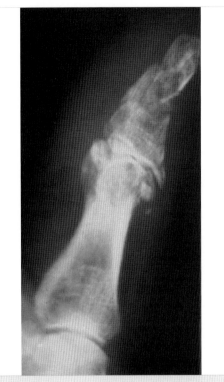

Fig. 5.5 Distal phalanx shaft fracture of the thumb, complex.

5.2.3 Extra-articular Fractures of the Distal Phalanx, Proximal

Table 5.3 Proximal extra-articular distal phalanx fractures

Fracture type	Surgical management	Procedure reference
Proximal extra-articular (▶ Fig. 5.6) AO: 7 1 to 5 3.2-B1/B2	Conservative: External splinting, percutaneous Kirschner wire occasionally	See Chapter 10.13.2

5.2.4 Intra-articular Fractures of the Distal Phalanx, Proximal

Table 5.4 Proximal intra-articular distal phalanx fractures

Fracture type	Surgical management	Procedure reference
Dorsal border AO: 7 1 to 5 3.1-C1 • Type I: small fragment without significant joint involvement / bony extensor tendon avulsion (▶ Fig. 5.7a) • Type II: fragment < 50% of the lateral joint line, joint congruent	Conservative: External splinting, e.g., stack splint 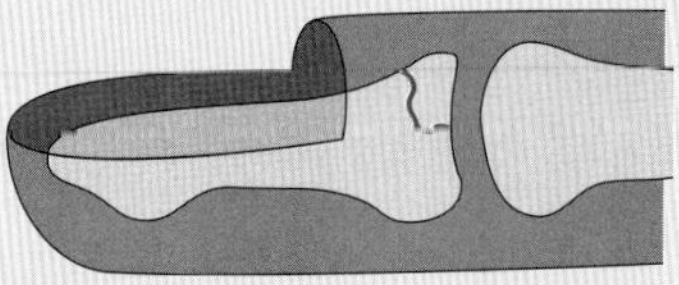	
	Refixation: Lengemann suture 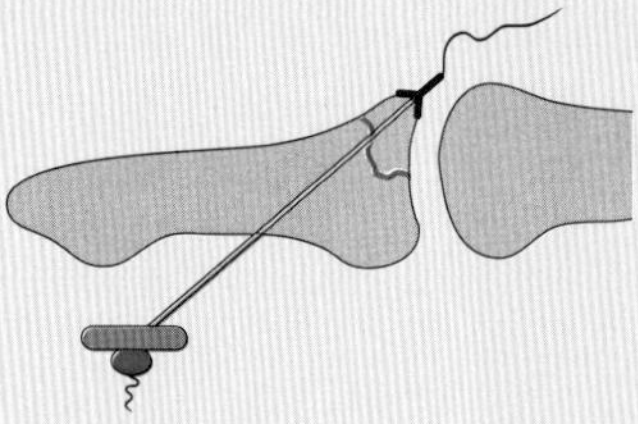	See Chapter 10.6.1
	With supporting tube 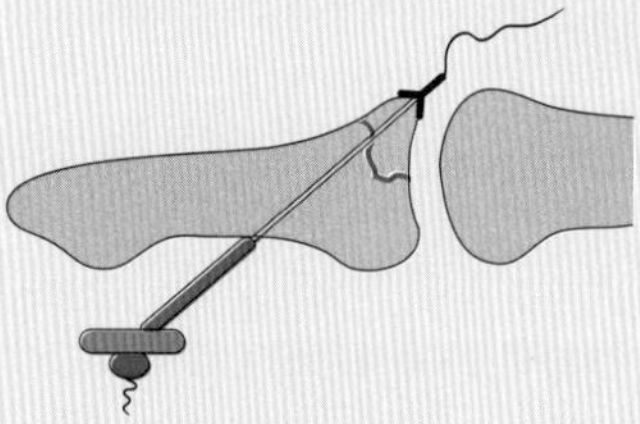	
	Ender/Hintringer method 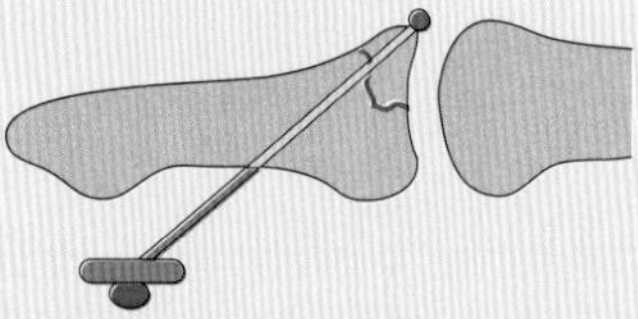	See Chapter 10.13.3
	Retrograde Kirschner wire 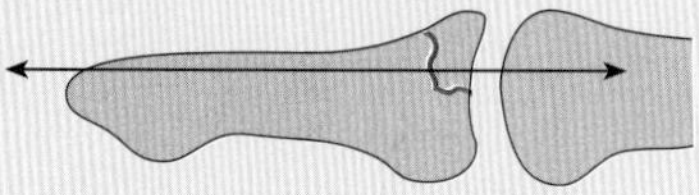	See Chapter 10.13.5
	Ishiguro operation 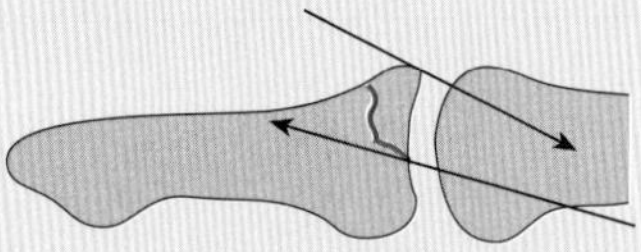	See Chapter 10.13.6
• Type III: fragment size at least 50% of the lateral joint line; intra-articular fracture with subluxation, especially in hyperextension (▶ Fig. 5.7b)	Screw (Kirschner wire) 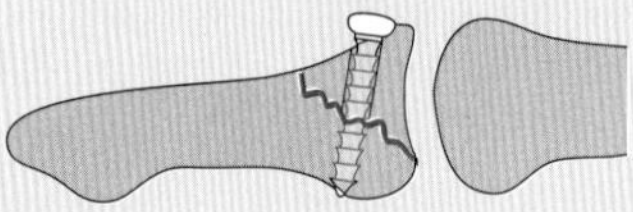	See Chapter 10.4.1

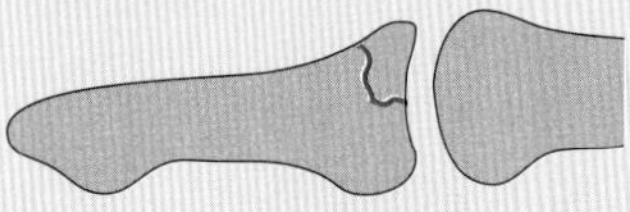

Table 5.4 (*Continued*)

Fracture type	Surgical management	Procedure reference
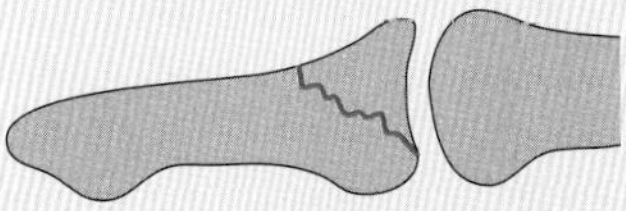 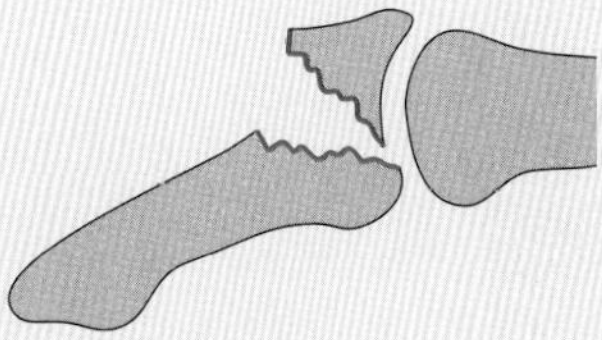	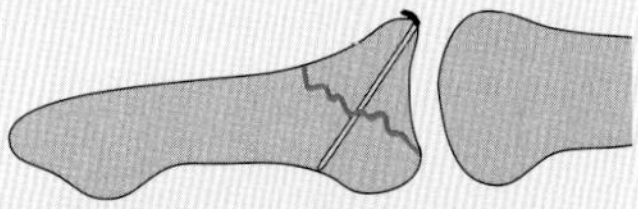	See Chapter 10.13.3
	Tension band wiring 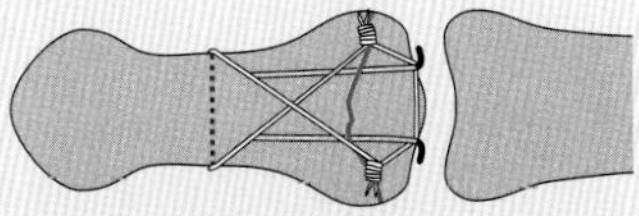 	See Chapter 10.13.1
	Hooked/pronged plate 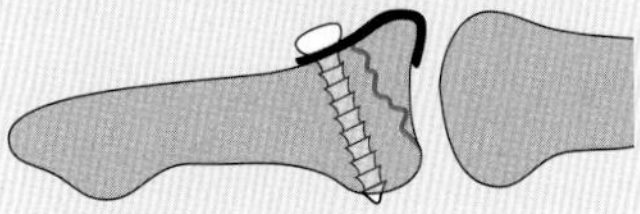 	See Chapter 10.17.1 Caution: nail matrix
Lateral border AO: 7 1 to 5 3.1-C1 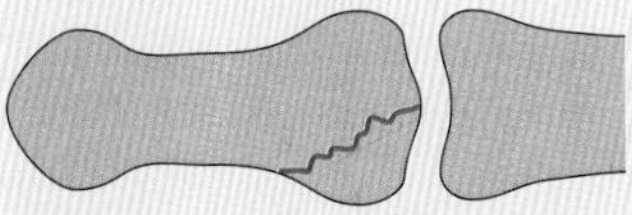 	Conservative: External splinting, e.g., stack splint 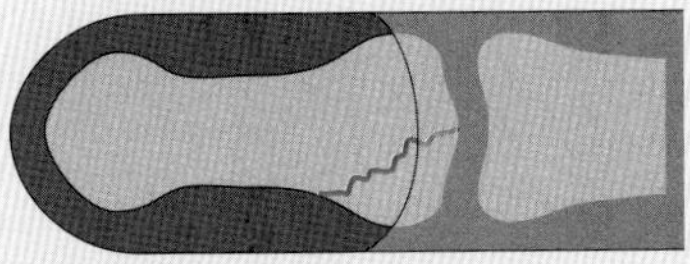 	See Chapter 10.13.2
	Refixation: Percutaneous Kirschner wire 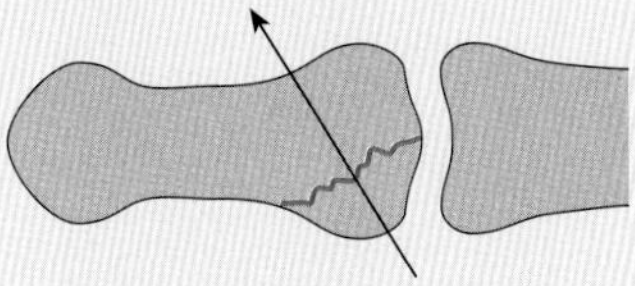 	See Chapter 10.13.2
	Lengemann suture 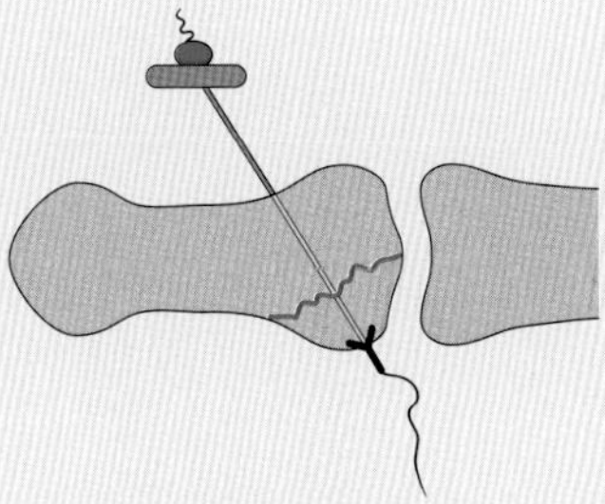 	See Chapter 10.16
	Ender/Hintringer method 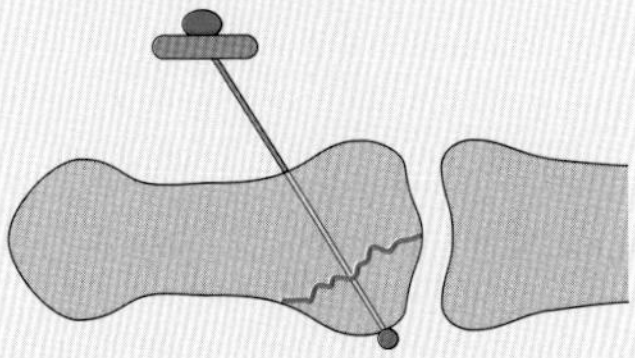 	See Chapter 10.13.3
	Screw 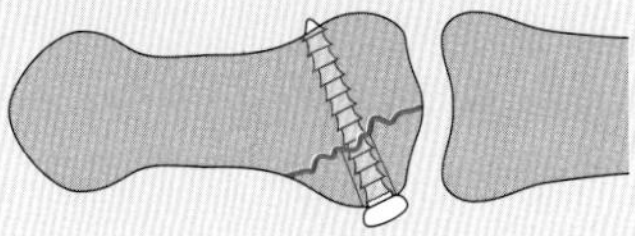 	See Chapter 10.4.1

Continued ▶

Table 5.4 (*Continued*)

Fracture type	Surgical management	Procedure reference
Palmar border (▶ Fig. 5.8) AO: 7 1 to 5 3.1-C1 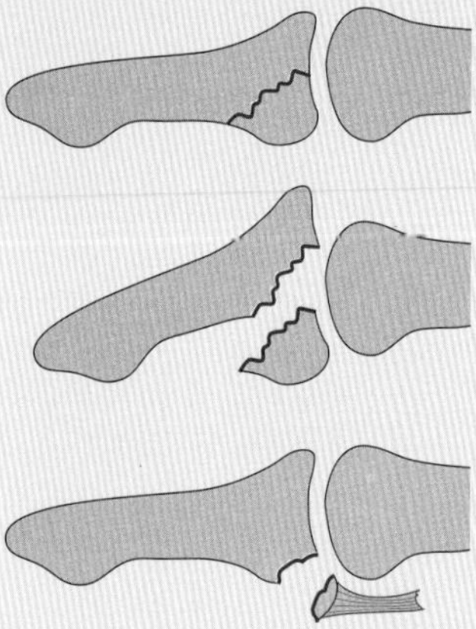	Ender/Hintringer method 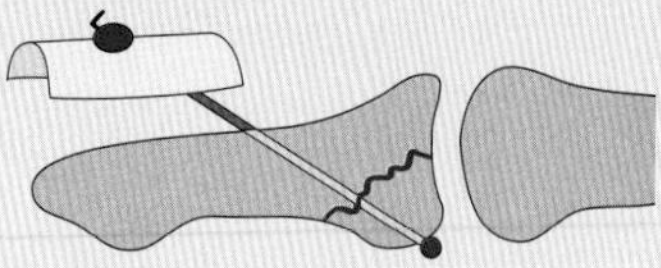	See Chapter 10.13.3
	Lengemann suture 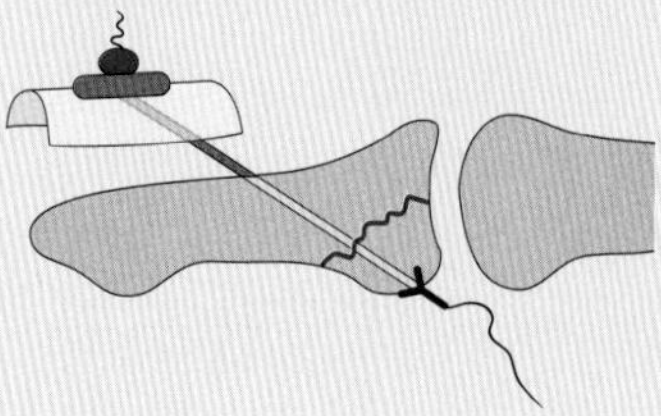	See Chapter 10.16
	Screw 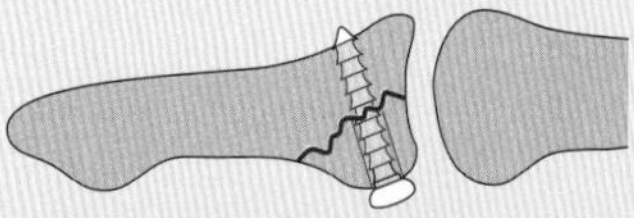	See Chapter 10.4.1
Depression AO: 7 1 to 5 3.1-C3 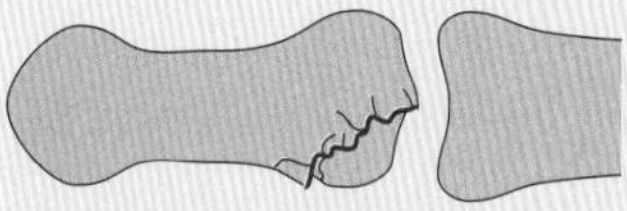	Elevation and Kirschner wire support (see depressed fracture of base of middle phalanx) 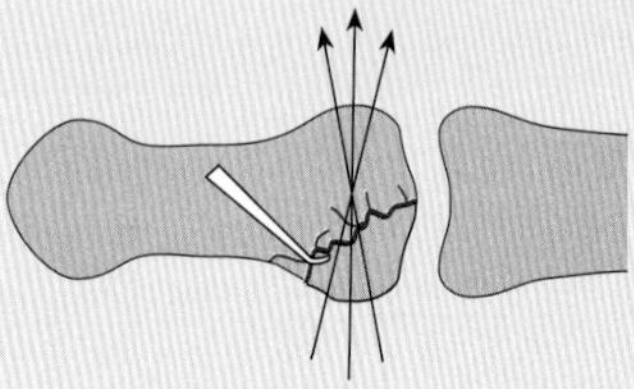	See Chapter 10.13.4
Complex (▶ Fig. 5.9) AO: 7 1 to 5 3.1-C3 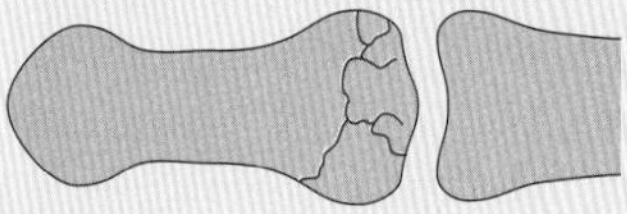	External fixator joint -bridging from dorsolateral, lateral 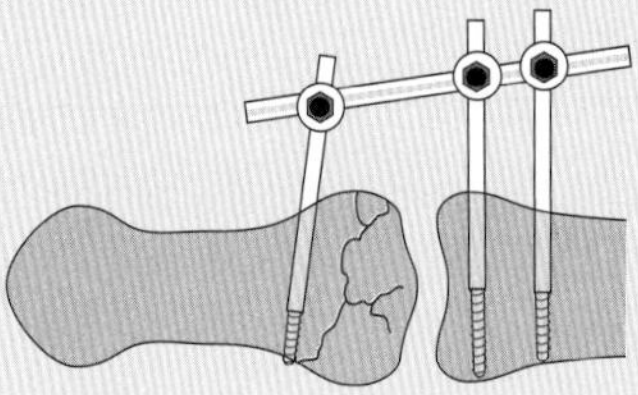	See Chapter 10.12.3

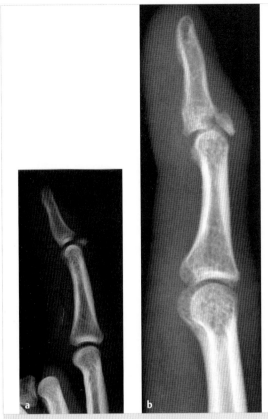

Fig. 5.7 Intra-articular distal phalanx fractures, proximal. Dorsal border. (a) Without dislocation, type I. (b) With minimal palmar subluxation, type II to III.

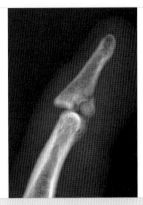

Fig. 5.8 Intra-articular distal phalanx fracture, proximal. Palmar border with dorsal dislocation, type II to III.

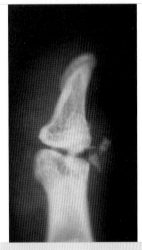

Fig. 5.9 Intra-articular distal phalanx fracture of the thumb, proximal, complex. Depression, posterolateral border.

5.3 Middle Phalanx and Proximal Phalanx Fractures

5.3.1 Intra-articular Fractures of the Middle/Proximal Phalanx, Distal

Table 5.5 Distal intra-articular middle/proximal phalanx fractures

Fracture type	Surgical management	Procedure reference
Monocondylar (▶ Fig. 5.10) AO: 7 1 to 5 1/2.3-C1 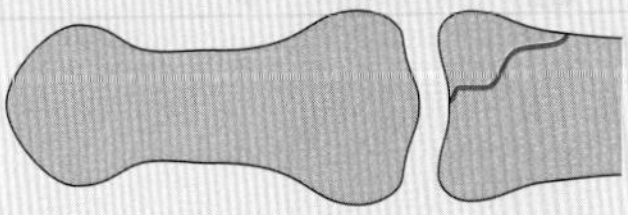	Percutaneous Kirschner wire 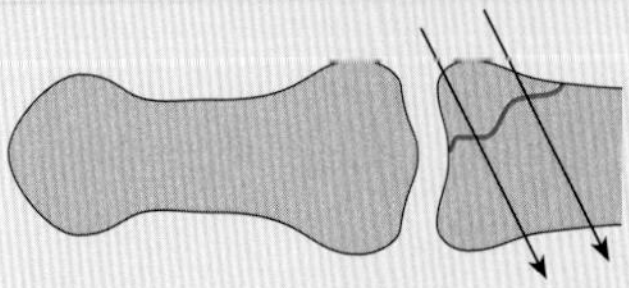	See Chapter 10.13.2
	Lag screw, correct size 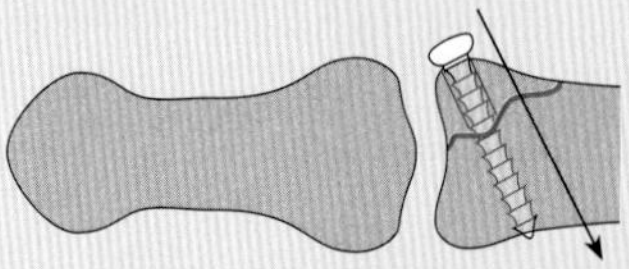	See Chapter 10.4.1
	Combination of lag screw and neutralization plate 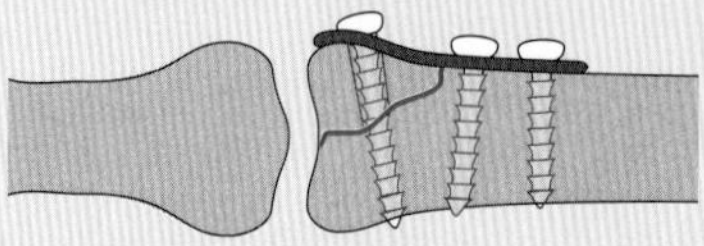	See Chapter 10.5.1
Bicondylar (▶ Fig. 5.11) AO: 7 1 to 5 1/2.3-C2 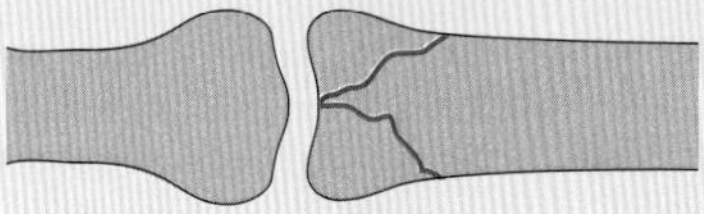	Percutaneous Kirschner wire 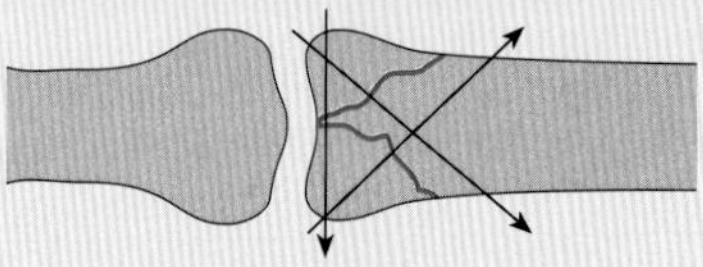	See Chapter 10.13.2
	Lag screws, correct size 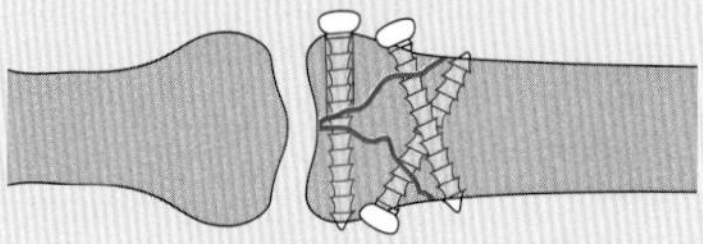	See Chapter 10.4.1
	Combination of lag screw and Kirschner wire 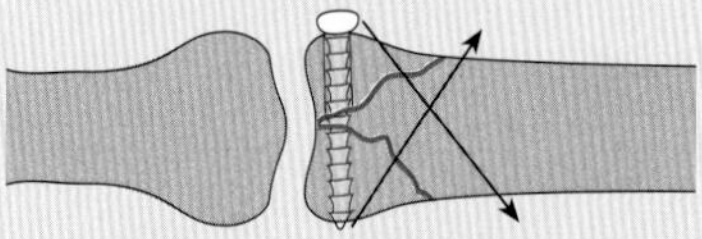	See Chapter 10.4.1, Chapter 10.13.2
Complex (▶ Fig. 5.12) AO: 7 1 to 5 1/2.3-C3 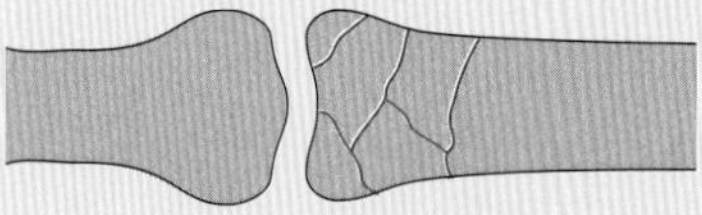	External fixator from dorsolateral, lateral 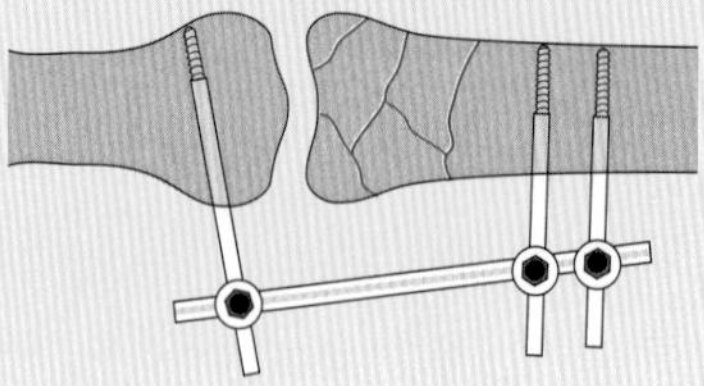	See Chapter 10.12.3

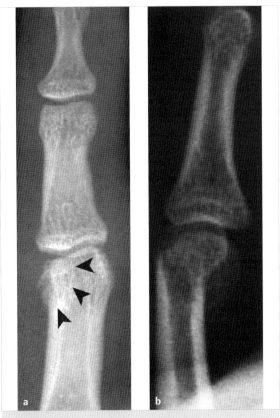

Fig. 5.10 Intra-articular proximal phalanx fracture, distal. X-ray in two planes (a,b).

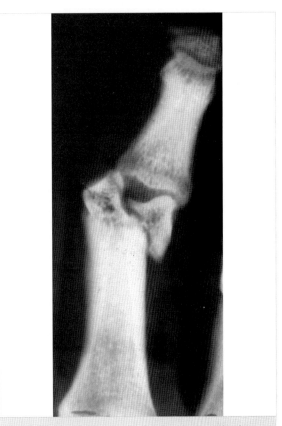

Fig. 5.11 Intra-articular proximal phalanx fracture, distal, bicondylar with misalignment.

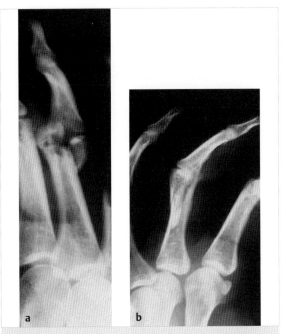

Fig. 5.12 Intra-articular proximal phalanx fracture, distal, complex. X-ray in two planes (a,b).

5.3.2 Extra-articular Fractures of the Middle/Proximal Phalanx, Distal

Table 5.6 Distal extra-articular middle/proximal phalanx fractures

Fracture type	Surgical management	Procedure reference
Transverse AO: 7 1 to 5 1/2.3-B1 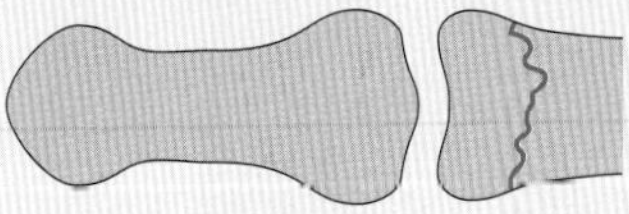	Percutaneous Kirschner wire 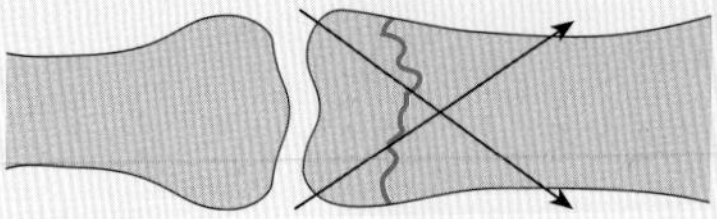	See Chapter 10.13.2
	Wire suture 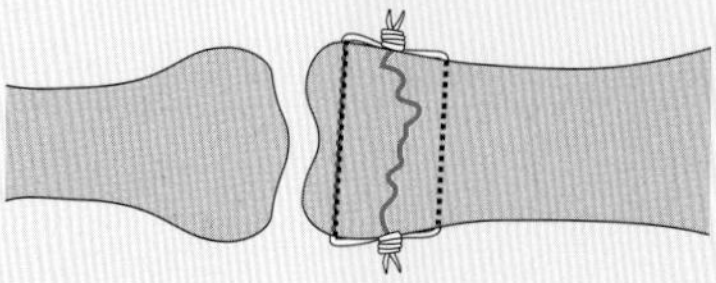	See Chapter 10.2.1
	Intramedullary pinning, antegrade or retrograde 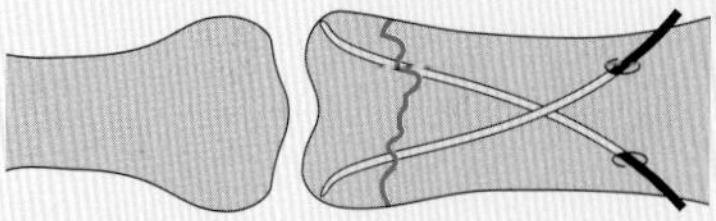	See Chapter 10.11.2, Chapter 10.11.3
	T-plate, H-plate 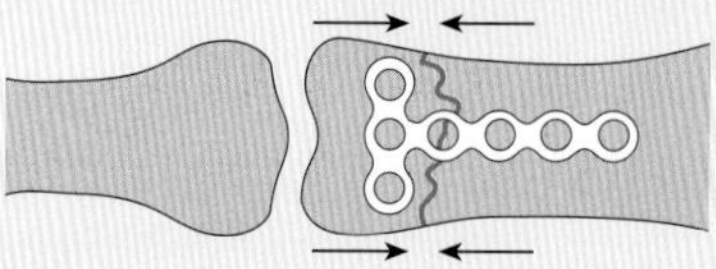	See Chapter 10.7.1
	Fixed-angle locking plate, correct size, possibly hybrid plate after interfragmentary compression 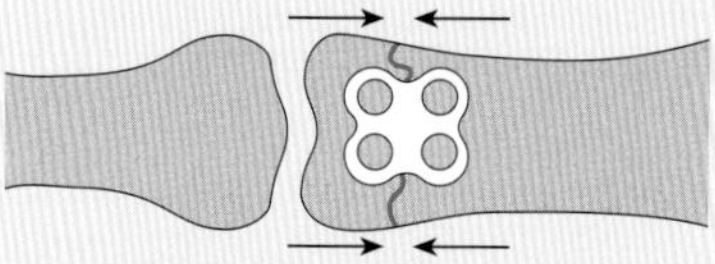	See Chapter 10.8.2 See Chapter 10.7.1
	Condylar plate, interfragmentary compression, possibly hybrid plate 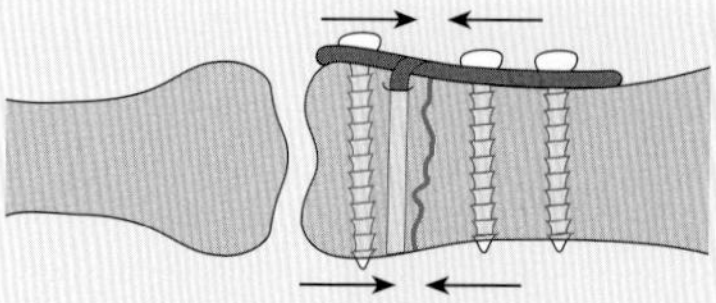	See Chapter 10.9.1 See Chapter 10.7.1
Spiral (▶ Fig. 5.13) AO: 7 1 to 5 1/2.3-B1 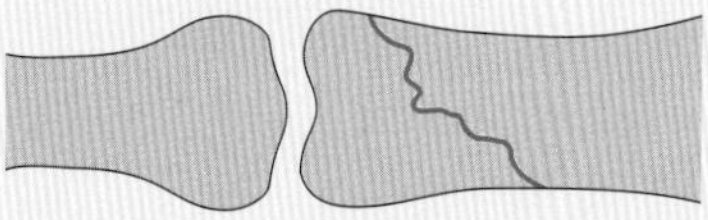	Percutaneous Kirschner wire 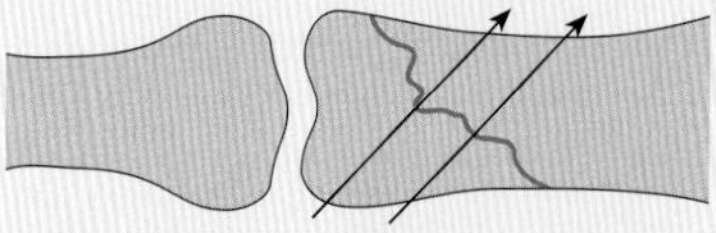	See Chapter 10.13.2
	Lag screw(s), correct size 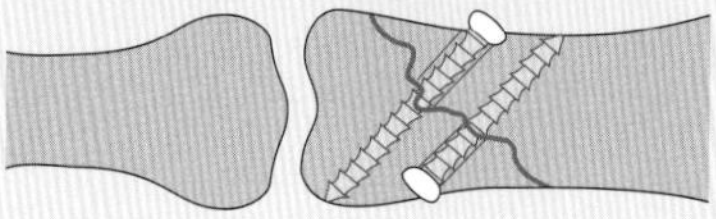	See Chapter 10.4.1

Table 5.6 (*Continued*)

Fracture type	Surgical management	Procedure reference
	Combination of lag screw and neutralization plate 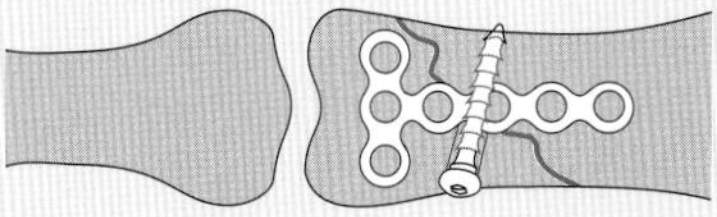	See Chapter 10.5.1
Complex (▶ Fig. 5.14) AO: 7 1 to 5 1/2.3-B3 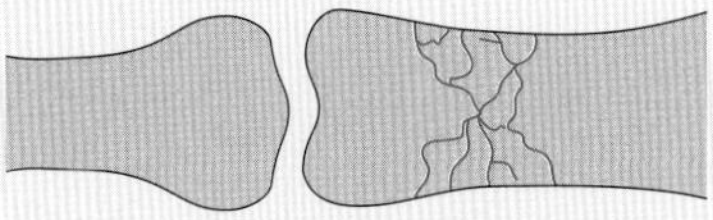	Fixed-angle locking plate 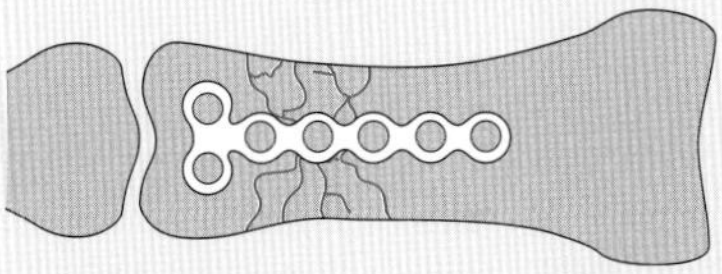	See Chapter 10.8.2
	External fixator 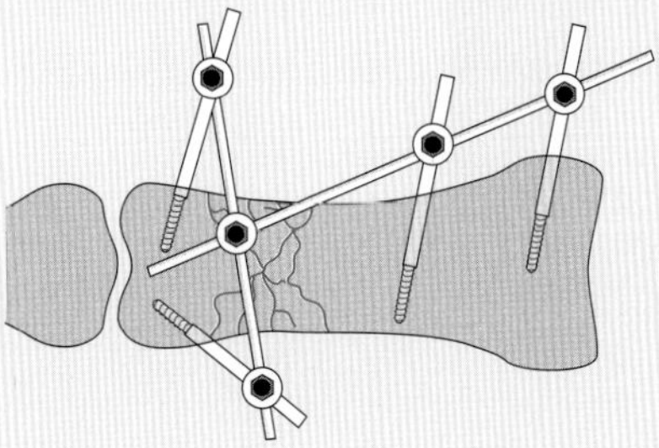	See Chapter 10.12.2, Chapter 10.12.3

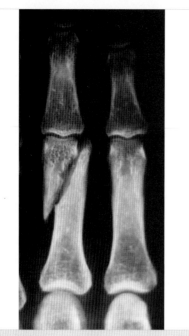

Fig. 5.13 Extra-articular proximal phalanx fracture, distal, spiral. Left middle finger.

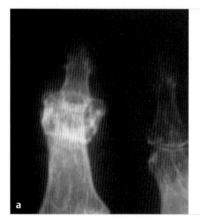
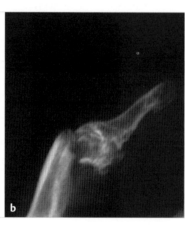

Fig. 5.14 Extra-articular middle phalanx fracture, distal, complex. X-ray in two planes (a,b).

5.3.3 Fractures of the Middle/Proximal Phalanx Shaft

Table 5.7 Middle/proximal phalanx shaft fractures

Fracture type	Surgical management	Procedure reference
Transverse (▶ Fig. 5.15) AO: 7 1 to 5 1/2.2-A1 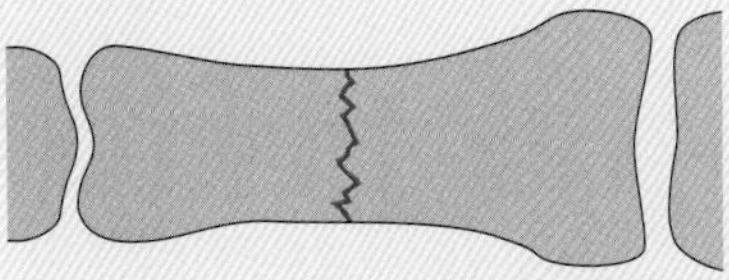	Wire suture (possibly with Kirschner wire) 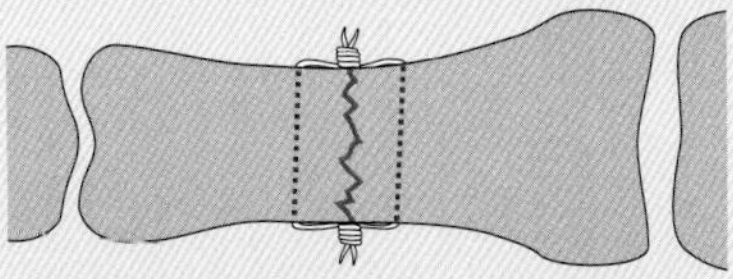	See Chapter 10.2.1
	Tension band wiring 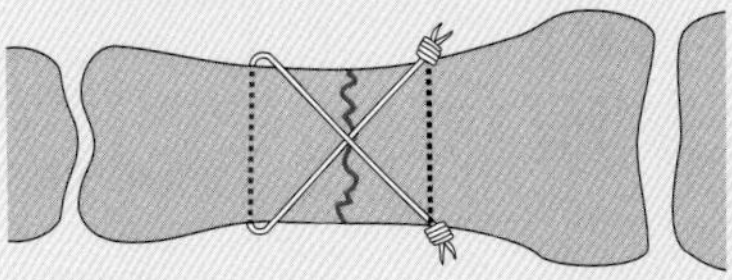	See Chapter 10.3.1
	Interfragmentary compression (straight plate, L-plate, H-plate, correct size) 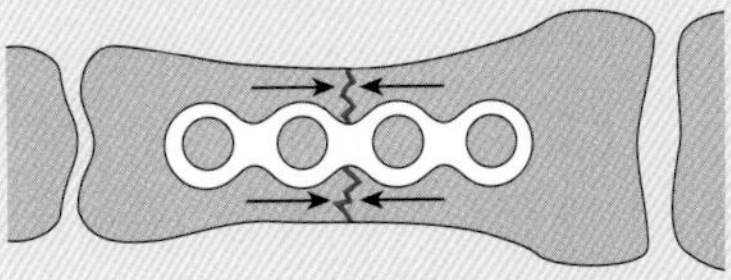	See Chapter 10.7.1
	Fixed-angle locking plate/hybrid plate after interfragmentary compression 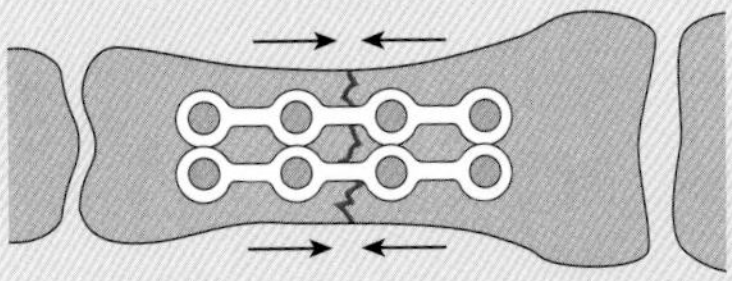	See Chapter 10.8.2
	Intramedullary pinning antegrade (retrograde) 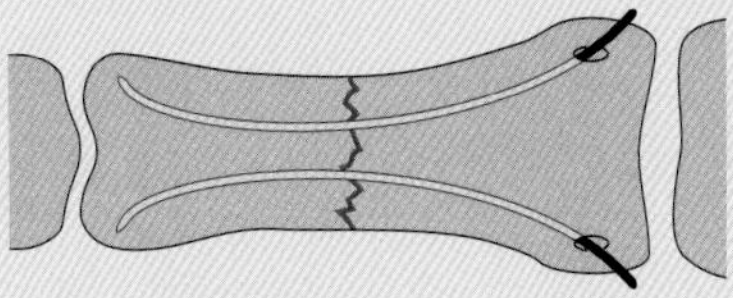	See Chapter 10.11.2
	Compression wire fixation 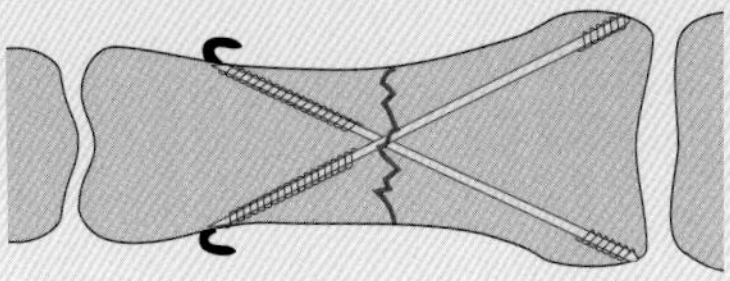	See Chapter 10.10.3

Continued ▶

Table 5.7 *(Continued)*

Fracture type	Surgical management	Procedure reference
Spiral (▶ Fig. 5.16) AO: 7 1 to 5 1/2.2-A1 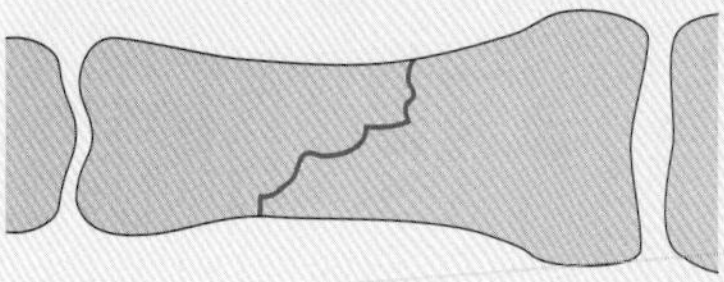	Lag screws, correct size 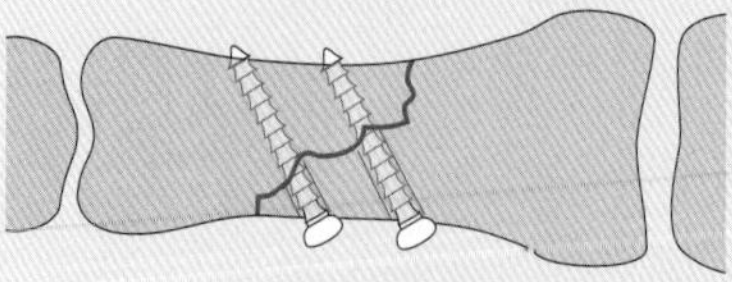	See Chapter 10.4.1
	Combination of lag screw and neutralization plate 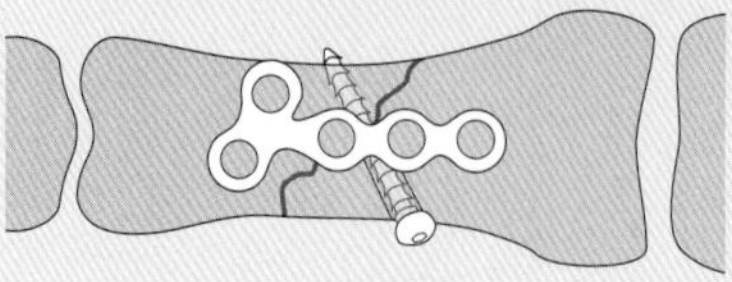	See Chapter 10.5.1
Complex (▶ Fig. 5.17 and ▶ Fig. 5.18) AO: 7 1 to 5 1/2.2-A3 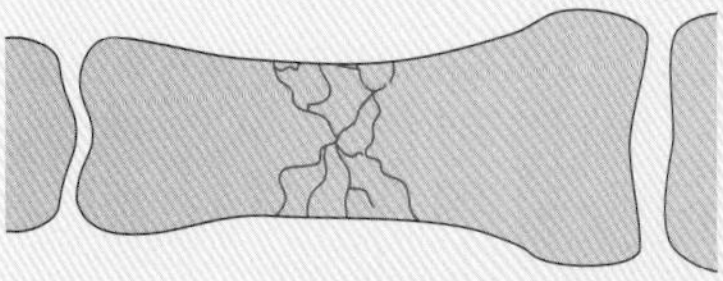	Fixed-angle locking plate 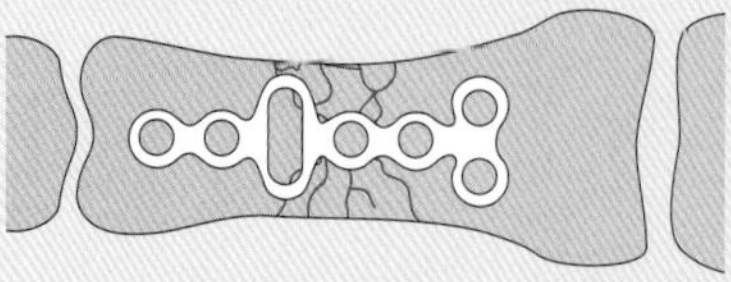	See Chapter 10.8.2
	External fixator 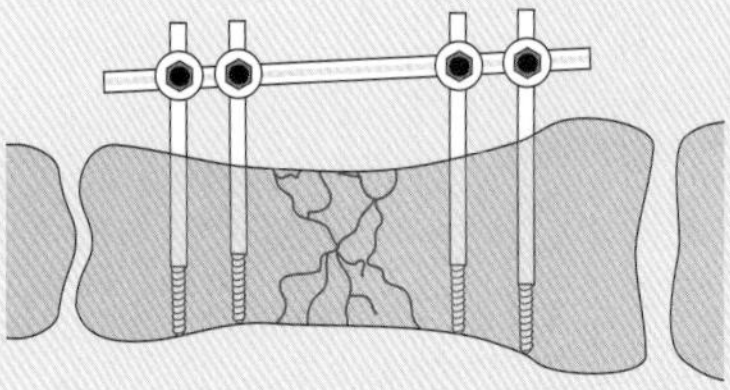	See Chapter 10.12.2, Chapter 10.12.3

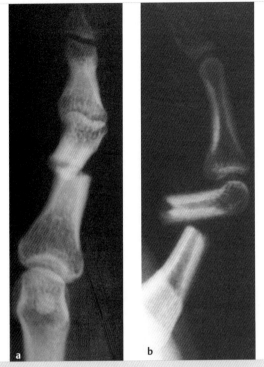

Fig. 5.15 Proximal phalanx shaft fracture, transverse. X-ray in two planes (a,b).

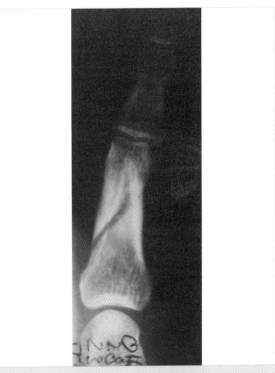

Fig. 5.16 Proximal phalanx shaft fracture, spiral.

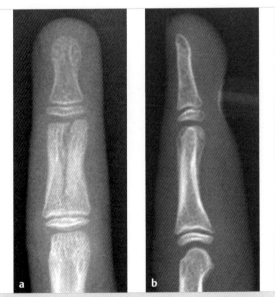

Fig. 5.17 Middle phalanx shaft fracture, complex. An 11-year-old child with crush injury from a bowling ball. X-ray in two planes (a,b).

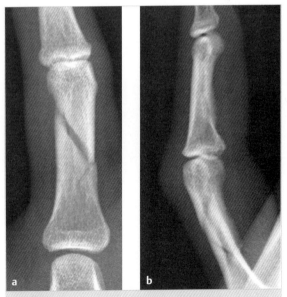

Fig. 5.18 Proximal phalanx shaft fracture, complex. X-ray in two planes (a,b).

5.3.4 Extra-articular Fractures of the Middle/Proximal Phalanx, Proximal

Table 5.8 Proximal extra-articular middle/proximal phalanx fractures

Fracture type	Surgical management	Procedure reference
Transverse (▶ Fig. 5.19) AO: 7 1 to 5 1/2.1-B1 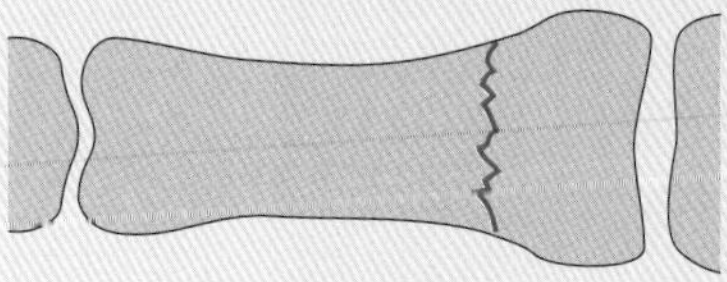	Percutaneous Kirschner wire 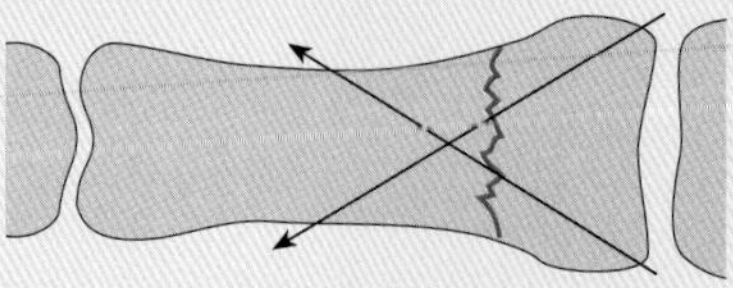	See Chapter 10.13.2
	Wire suture (possibly with Kirschner wire) 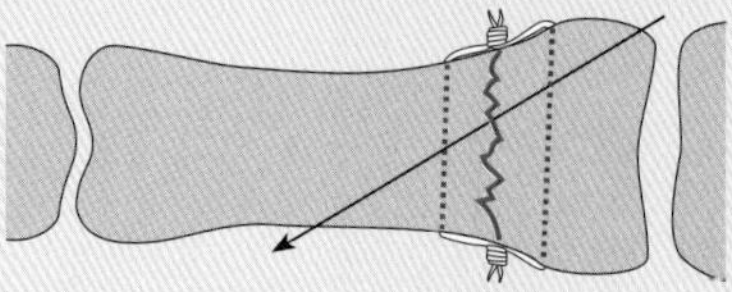	See Chapter 10.2.1
	Compression plate (T-plate, L-plate, H-plate) 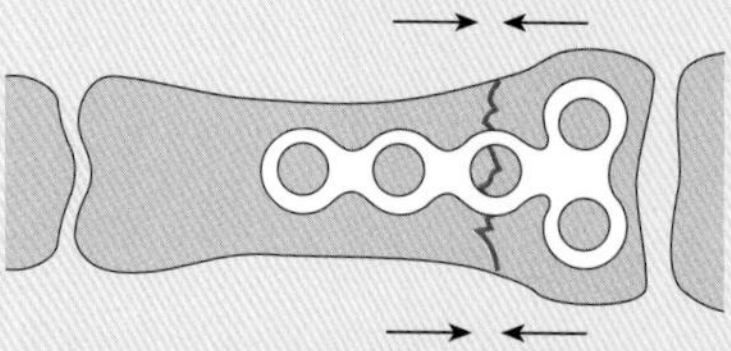	See Chapter 10.7.1
	Fixed-angle locking plate/hybrid-plate after interfragmentary compression 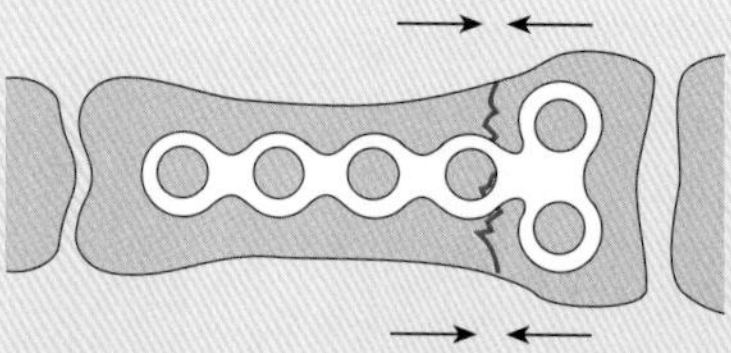	See Chapter 10.8.2 See Chapter 10.7.1
	Retrograde intramedullary Kirschner wire splinting/ pinning 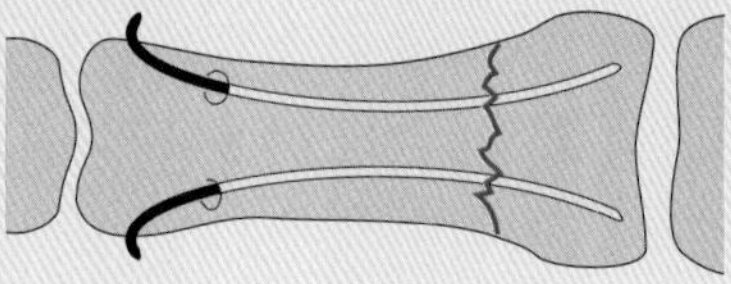	See Chapter 10.11.3

Table 5.8 (*Continued*)

Fracture type	Surgical management	Procedure reference
Spiral (▶ Fig. 5.20) AO: 7 1 to 5 1/2.1-B1 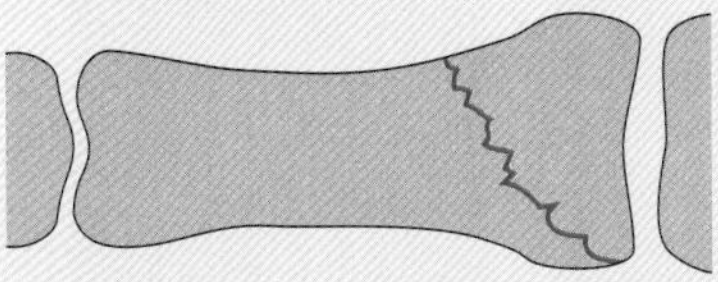	Percutaneous Kirschner wire 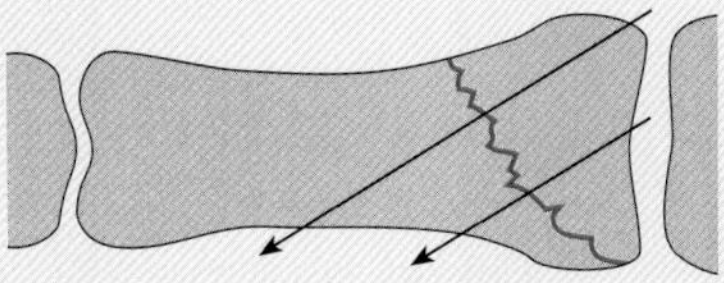	See Chapter 10.13.2
	Lag screw (s), correct size 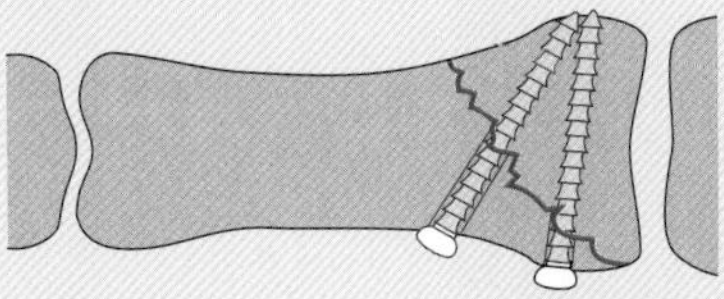	See Chapter 10.4.1
	Combination of lag screw and neutralization plate 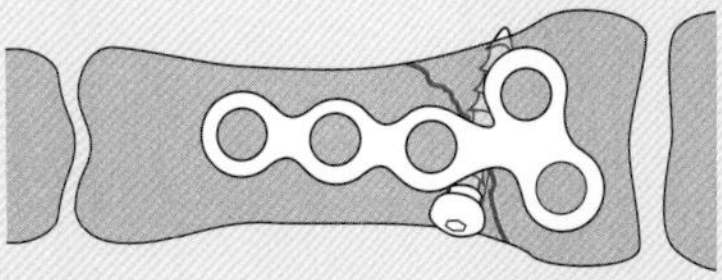	See Chapter 10.5.1
Complex (▶ Fig. 5.21) AO: 7 1 to 5 1/2.1-B3 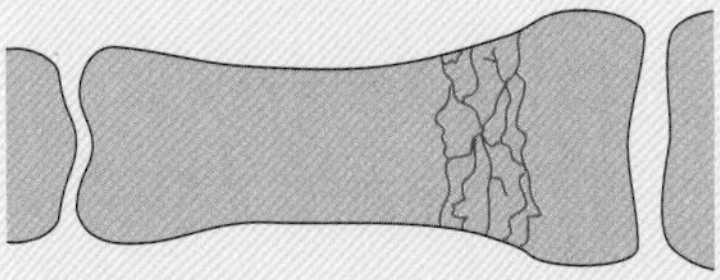	Fixed-angle locking plate/hybrid plate 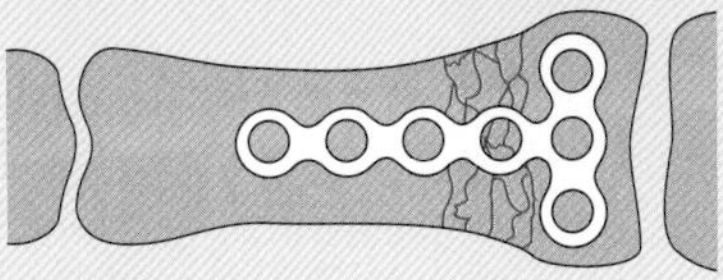	See Chapter 10.8.2
	External fixator 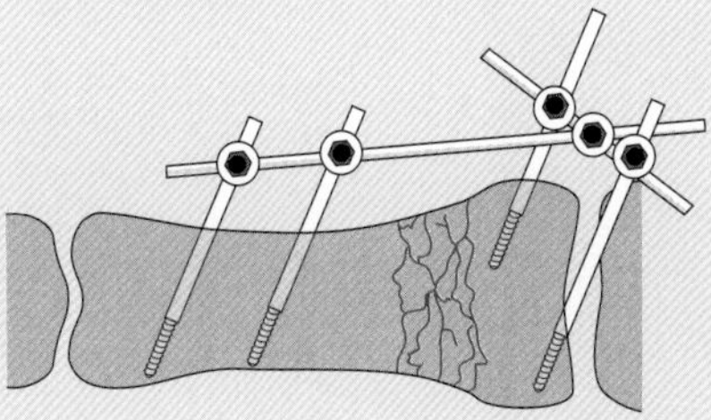	See Chapter 10.12.2, Chapter 10.12.3

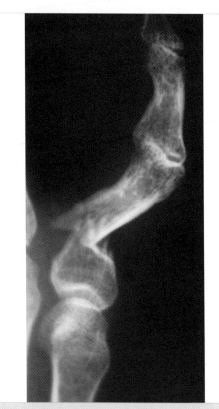

Fig. 5.19 Extra-articular proximal phalanx fracture, proximal, transverse. Right fifth finger.

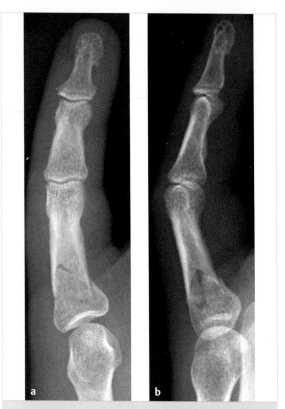

Fig. 5.20 Extra-articular proximal phalanx fracture, proximal, spiral. Left fifth finger, X-ray in two planes (a,b).

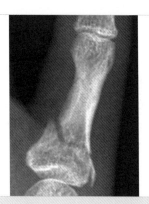

Fig. 5.21 Extra-articular proximal phalanx fracture, proximal, complex.

5.3.5 Intra-articular Fractures of the Middle/Proximal Phalanx, Proximal

Table 5.9 Proximal intra-articular middle/proximal phalanx fractures

Fracture type	Surgical management	Procedure reference
Dorsal avulsion AO: 7 1 to 5 1/2.1-C1 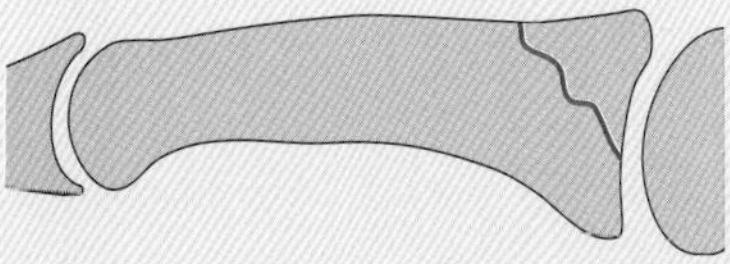	Percutaneous Kirschner wire 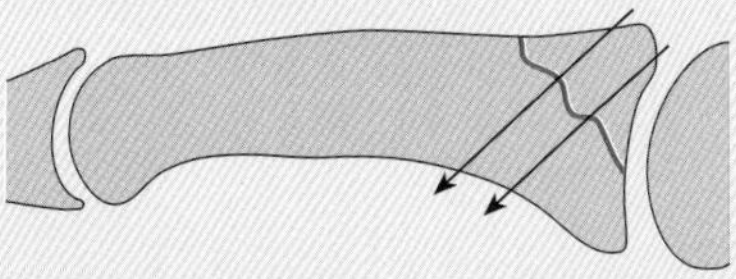	See Chapter 10.13.2
	Lag screw, correct size 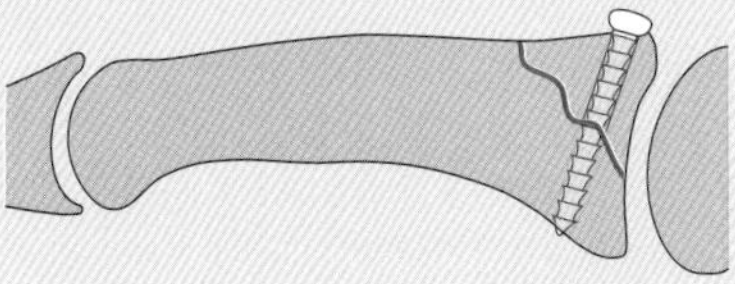	See Chapter 10.4.1
	(hooked/pronged plate) 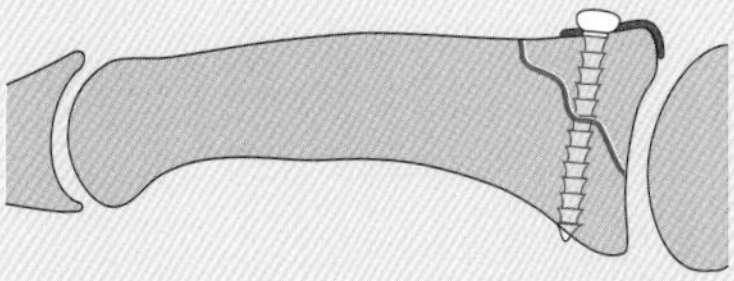	See Chapter 10.17.1
Lateral avulsion 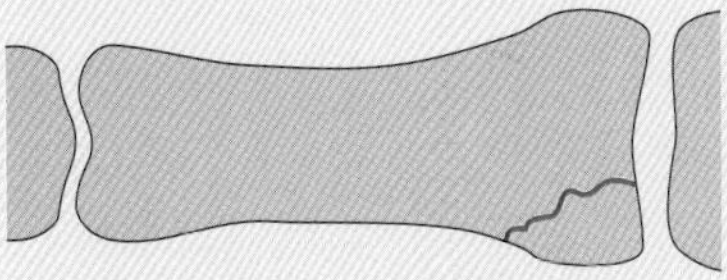	Percutaneous Kirschner wire 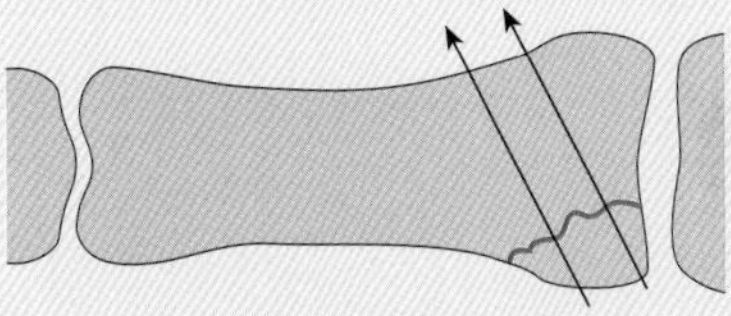	See Chapter 10.13.2
	Lag screw, correct size 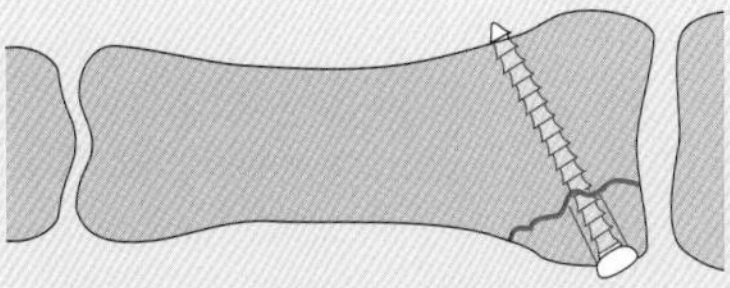	See Chapter 10.4.1
	(Lengemann suture) 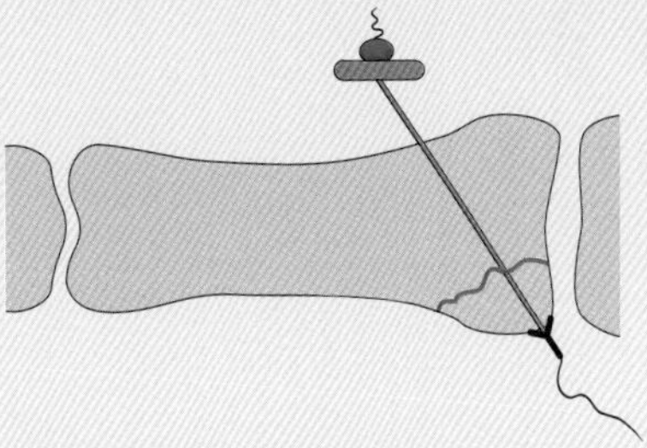	See Chapter 10.16.1
	Ender-Hintringer wire hook 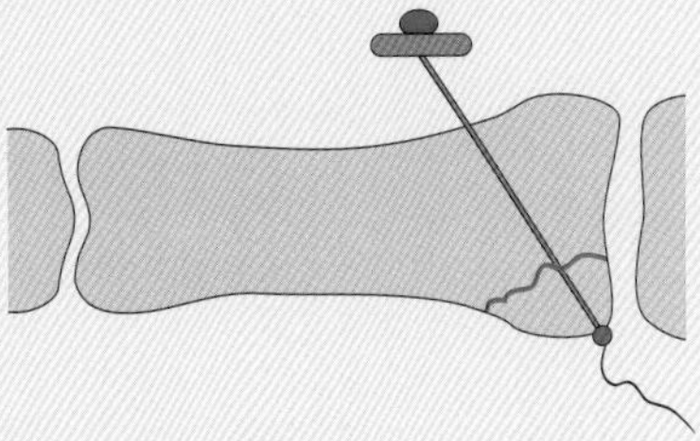	See Chapter 10.13.3

Continued ▶

Table 5.9 (*Continued*)

Fracture type	Surgical management	Procedure reference
Palmar avulsion (▶ Fig. 5.22, ▶ Fig. 5.23) 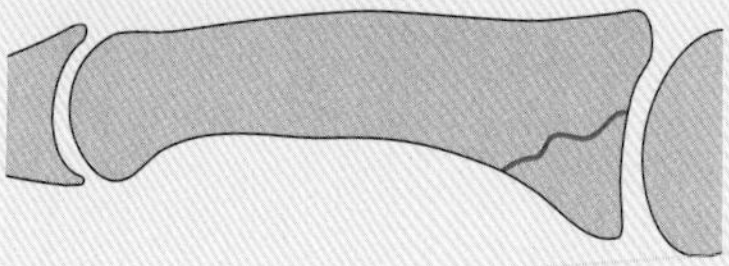	Lag screw, correct size from palmar 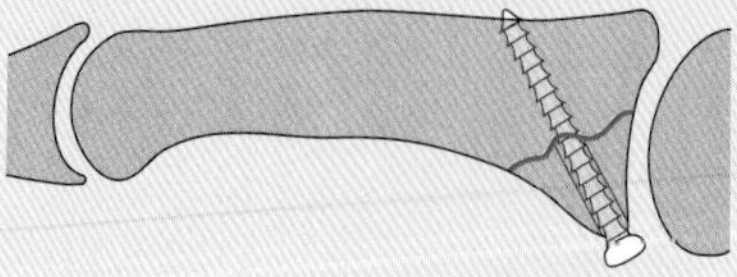	See Chapter 10.4.1
	Lag screw, correct size from dorsal 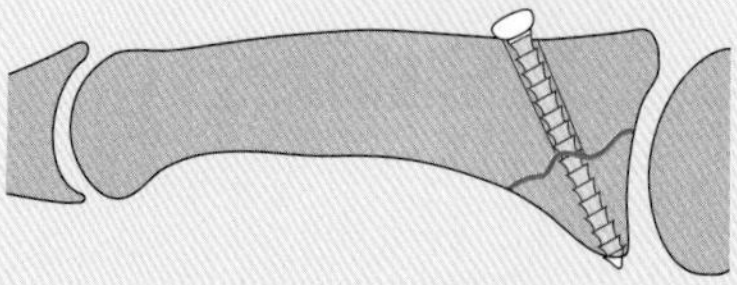	See Chapter 10.4.1
	Dynamic extension/traction after Suzuki and others Proximal interphalangeal joint 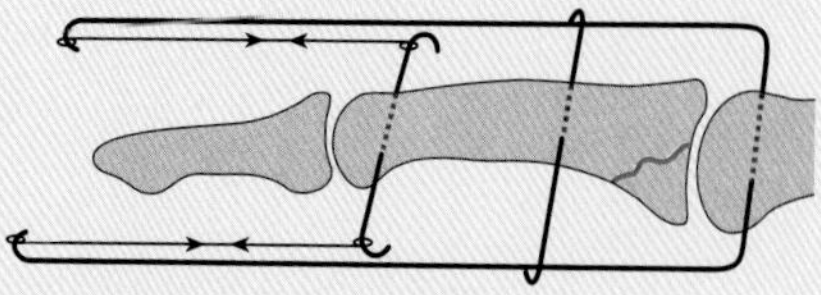	See Chapter 10.15.1
T, Y fracture AO: 7 1 to 5 1/2.1-C2 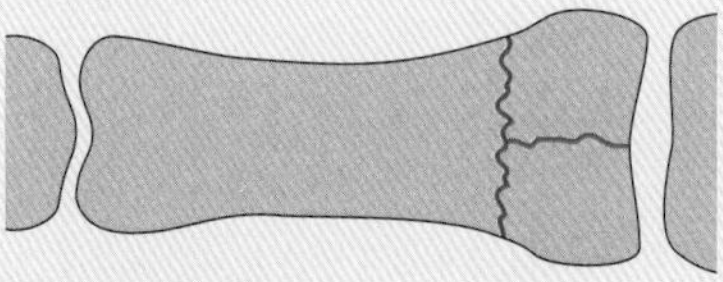 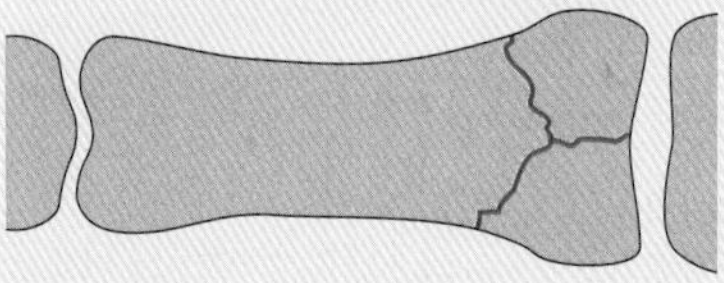	Percutaneous Kirschner wires 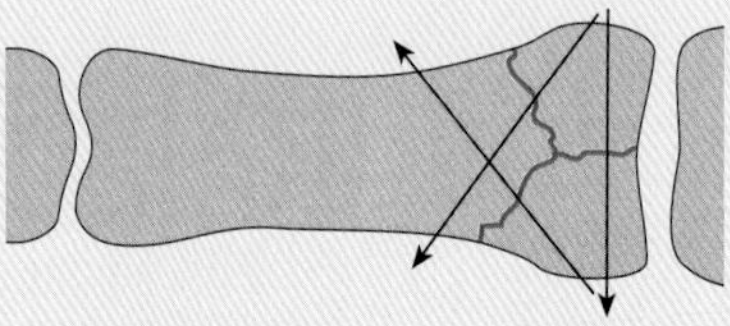	See Chapter 10.13.2
	Lag screw(s) 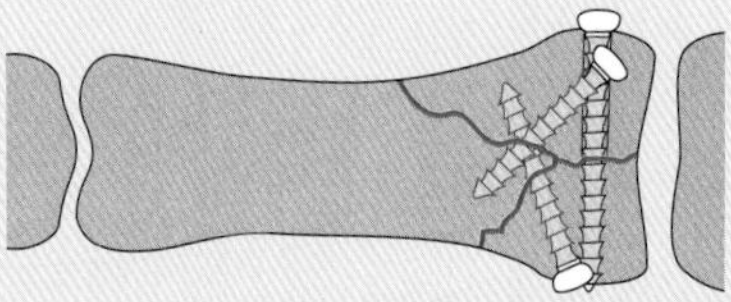	See Chapter 10.4.1
	Combination of lag screw and neutralization plate / protective plate 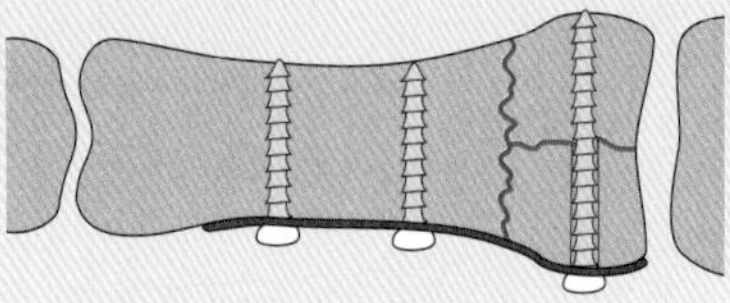	See Chapter 10.5.1

Table 5.9 (Continued)

Fracture type	Surgical management	Procedure reference
Depressed fracture AO: 7 1 to 5 1/2.1-C3 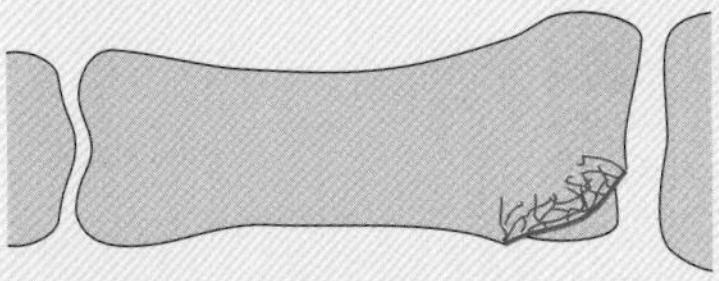	Ender–Hintringer "plugging" method 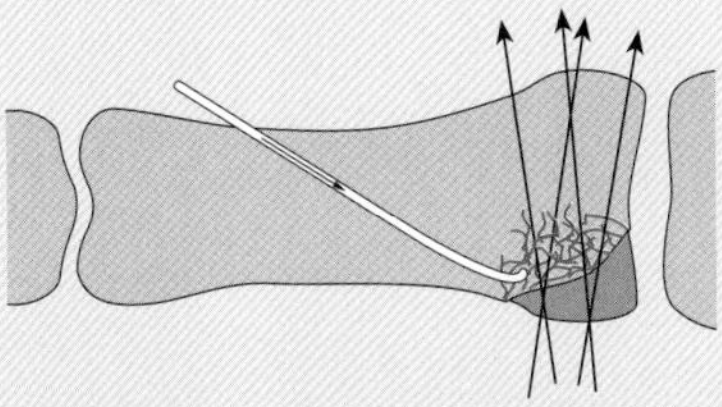	See Chapter 10.13.4
Complex (▶ Fig. 5.24, ▶ Fig. 5.25) AO: 7 1 to 5 1/2.1-C3 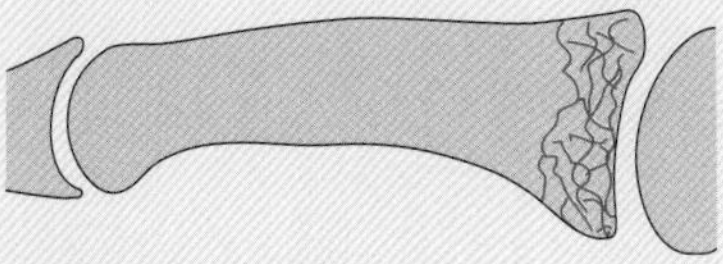	Joint-bridging external fixator / fixed-angle locking plate Flexion of 80° in MCPJ Maximum flexion of 30° in PIPJ 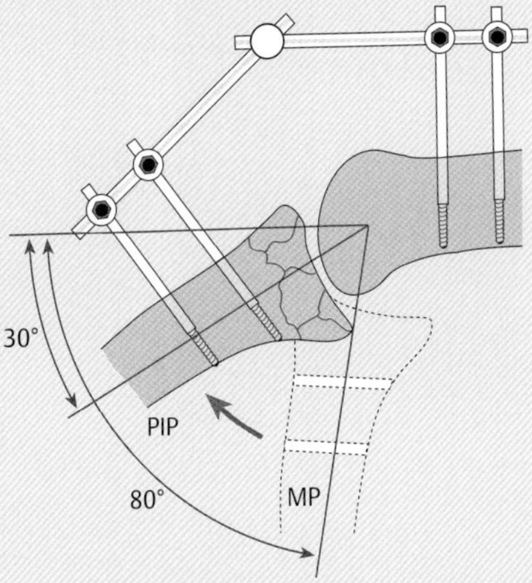	See Chapter 10.12.3, Chapter 10.8.2
	Dynamic extension/traction after Suzuki and others PIPJ 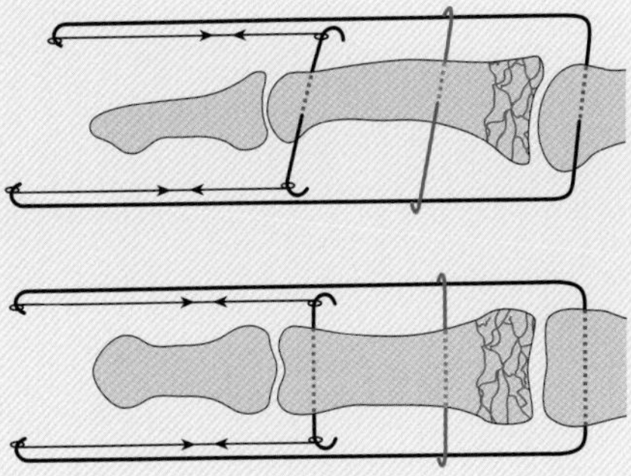	See Chapter 10.15.1

Abbreviations: MCPJ, metacarpophalangeal joint; PIPJ, proximal interphalangeal joint.

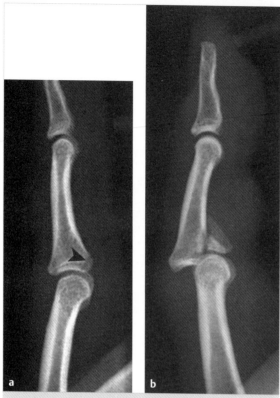

Fig. 5.22 Intra-articular middle phalanx fracture, proximal. (a) Bony avulsion of the palmar plate at the base of the middle phalanx. (b) Large palmar avulsion at the base of the middle phalanx with dorsal dislocation.

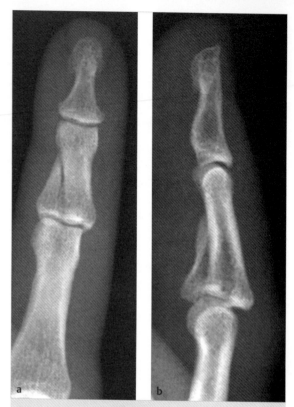

Fig. 5.23 Intra-articular spiral fracture at the base of the middle phalanx with dorsal dislocation. Right fifth finger, X-ray in two planes (a,b).

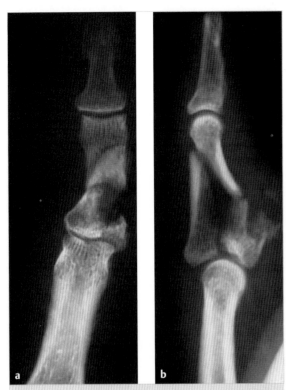

Fig. 5.24 Intra-articular middle phalanx fracture, proximal, complex. Multifragmentary fracture. X-ray in two planes (a,b).

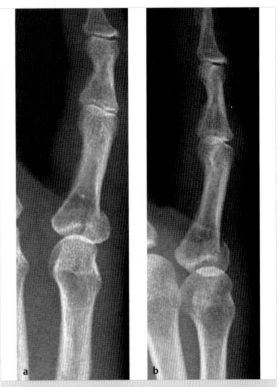

Fig. 5.25 Intra-articular fracture of the base of the proximal phalanx with depression. Left fifth finger, X-ray in two planes (a,b).

5.4 Metacarpal Fractures

5.4.1 Intra-articular Fractures of the Metacarpals, Distal

Table 5.10 Distal intra-articular metacarpal fractures

Fracture type	Surgical management	Procedure reference
Spiral, monocondylar (▶ Fig. 5.26) AO: 7 1 to 5 0.3-C1 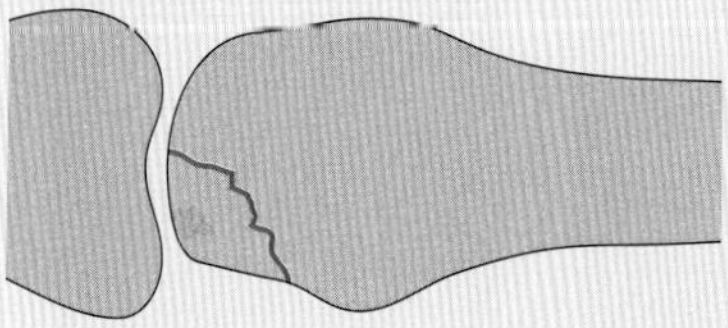	Percutaneous Kirschner wire 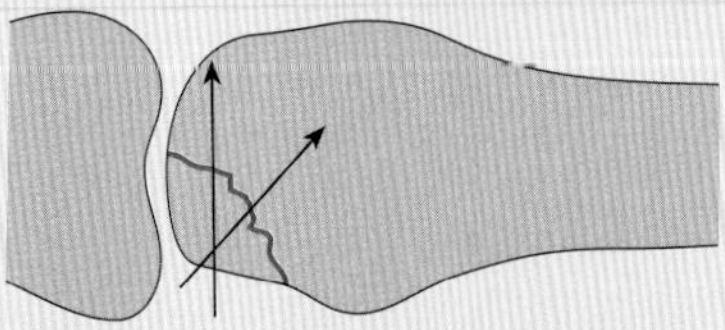	See Chapter 10.13.2
	Lag screw(s), correct size; if necessary, in combination with Kirschner wire 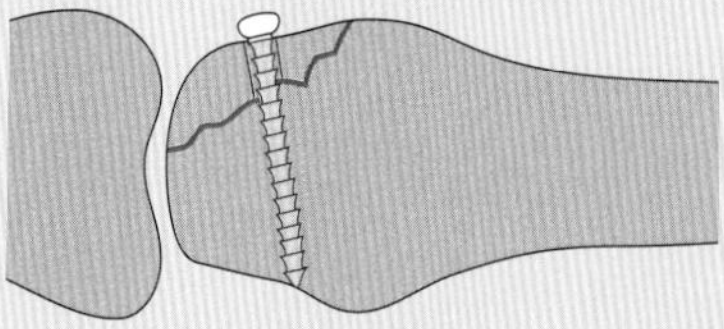	See Chapter 10.4.1, Chapter 10.6.1
T, Y fracture, bicondylar AO: 7 1 to 5 0.3-C2 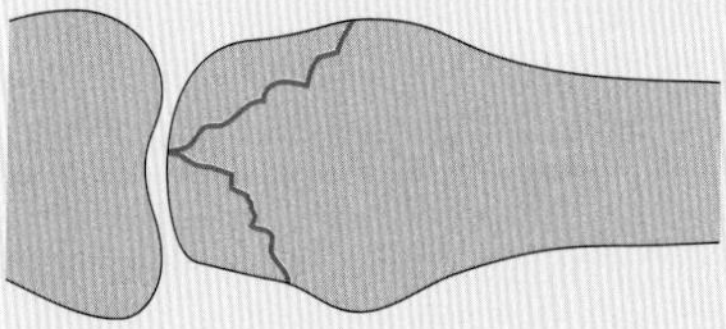 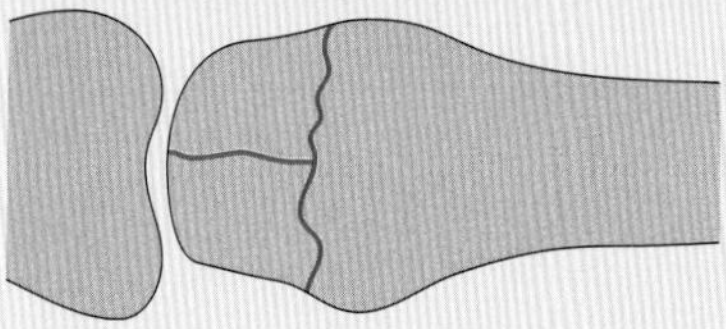	Lag screw(s), correct size, combination with Kirschner wire 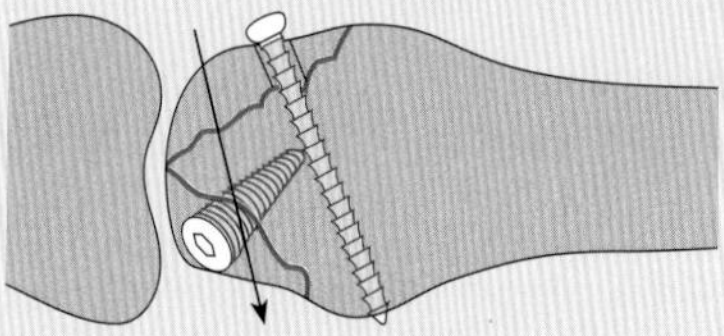 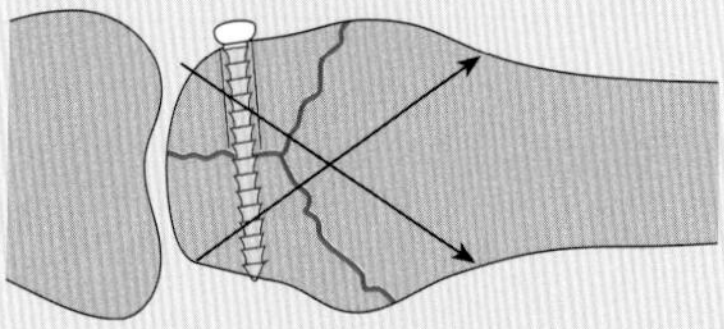	See Chapter 10.4.1, Chapter 10.6.1, Chapter 10.13.2
	Absorbable pins from the joint surface 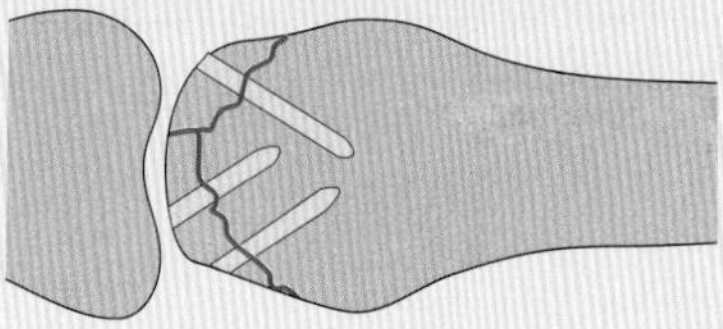	See Chapter 10.18

Table 5.10 (*Continued*)

Fracture type	Surgical management	Procedure reference
Complex (▶ Fig. 5.27) AO: 7 1 to 5 0.3-C3	Joint-bridging external fixator, metacarpophalangeal joint in 80° flexion	See Chapter 10.12.3

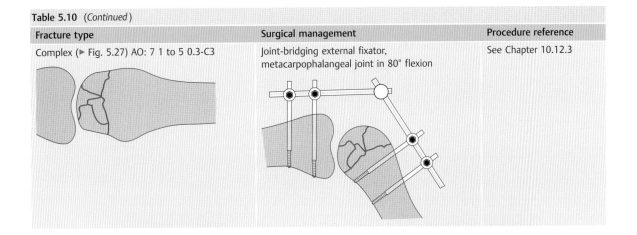

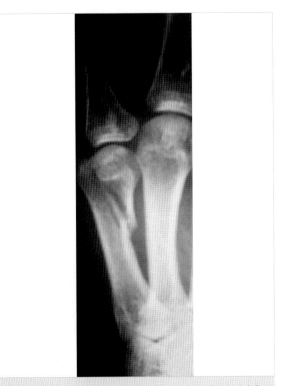

Fig. 5.26 Intra-articular metacarpal fracture, distal, spiral, left fifth finger.

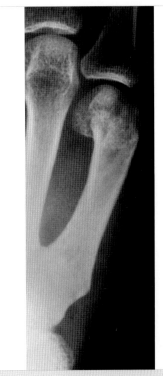

Fig. 5.27 Intra-articular metacarpal fracture, distal, complex, right fifth finger.

5.4.2 Extra-articular Fractures of the Metacarpals, Distal

Table 5.11 Distal extra-articular metacarpal fractures

Fracture type	Surgical management	Procedure reference
Transverse, simple (▶ Fig. 5.28) AO: 7 1 to 5 0.3-B1 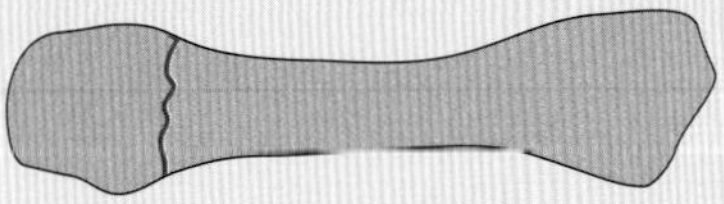	Intramedullary pinning from proximal 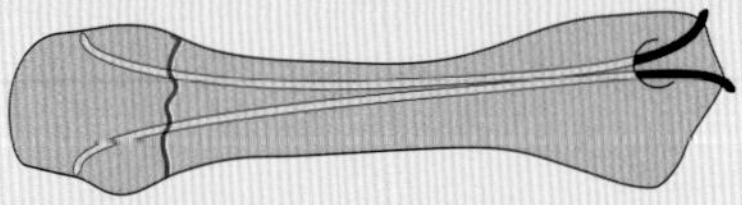	See Chapter 10.11.1
Transverse with third fragment AO: 7 1 to 5 0.3-B2 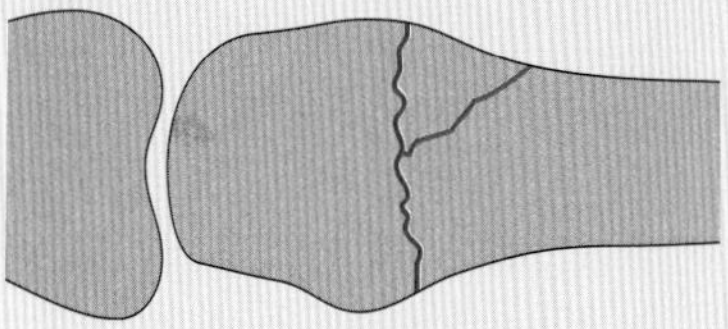	Wire suture, possibly plus Kirschner wire 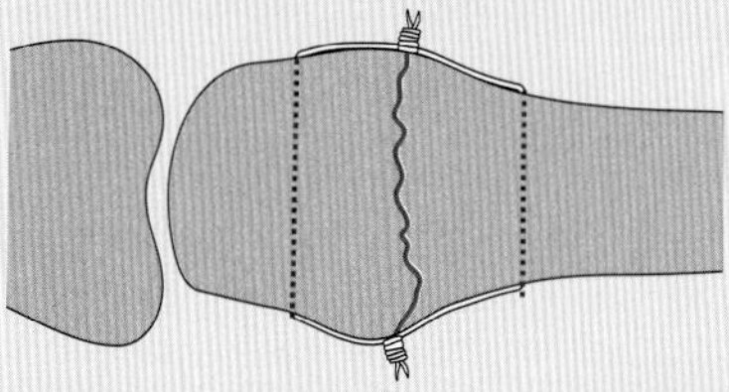	See Chapter 10.2.1
	Tension band wiring 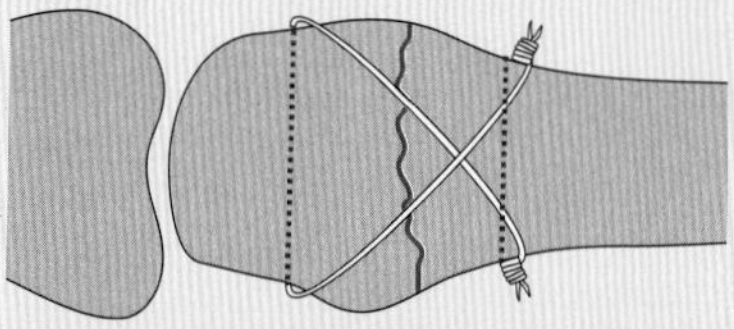	See Chapter 10.3.2
	Percutaneous Kirschner wires via condyles 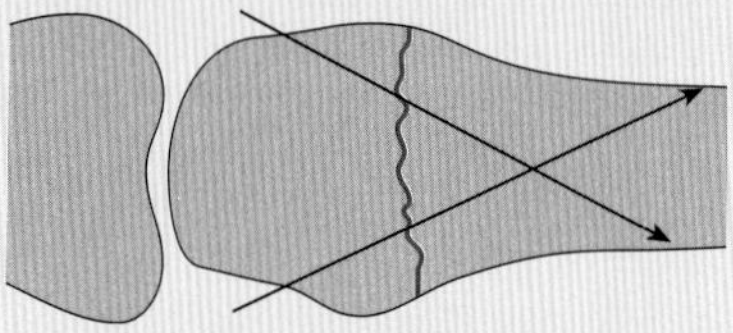	See Chapter 10.13.2
	Percutaneous transfixation 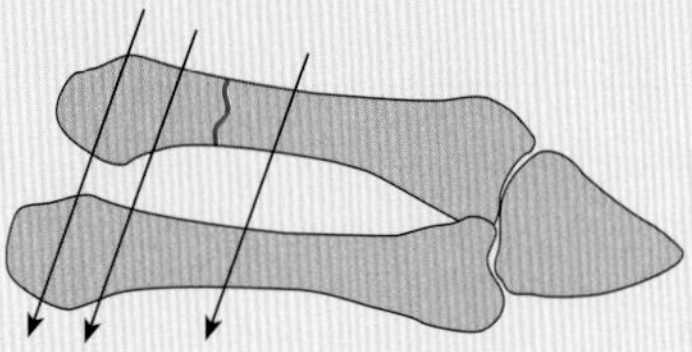	See Chapter 10.13.7

Table 5.11 (*Continued*)

Fracture type	Surgical management	Procedure reference
	Intramedullary pinning plus transfixation 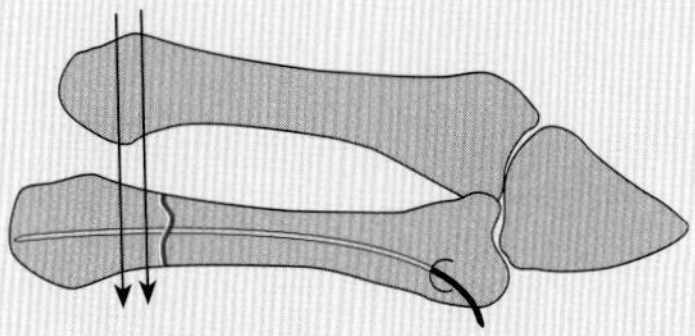	See Chapter 10.11.1, Chapter 10.13.7
	T-, L-, H-plate, fixed-angle locking plate/hybrid plate after interfragmentary compression 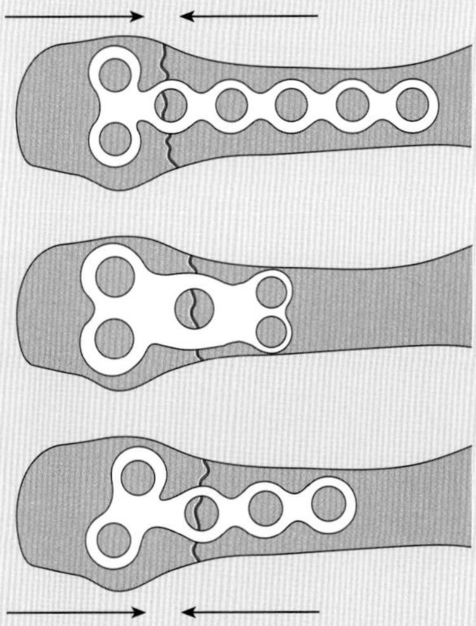	See Chapter 10.8.2, See Chapter 10.7.1
Spiral (▶ Fig. 5.29) AO: 7 1 to 5 0.3-B1 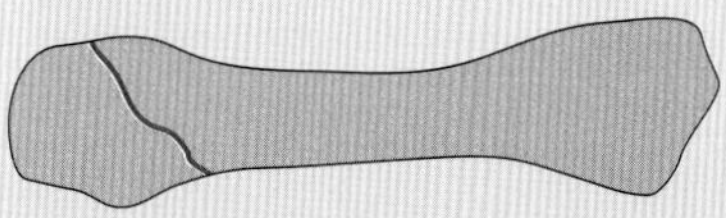	Intramedullary pinning from proximal 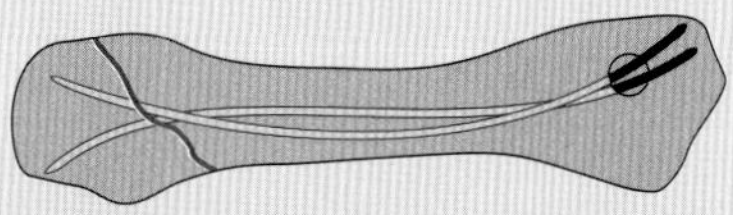	See Chapter 10.11.1
	Transcondylar percutaneous Kirschner wires from distal 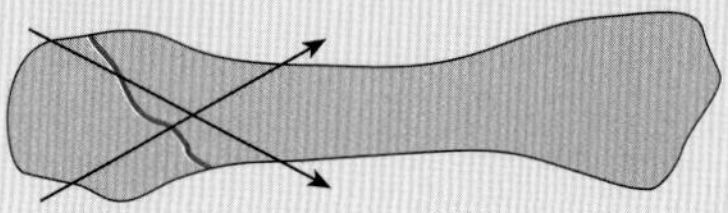	See Chapter 10.13.2
	Percutaneous transfixation 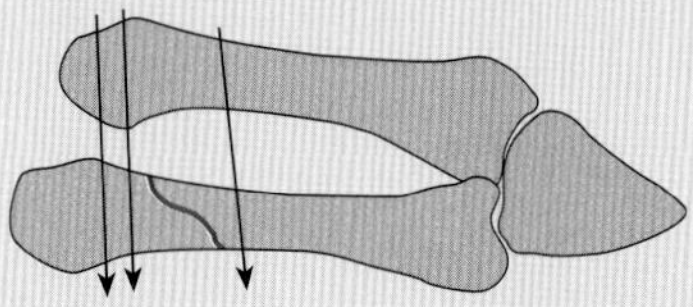	See Chapter 10.13.7
	Lag screw(s) 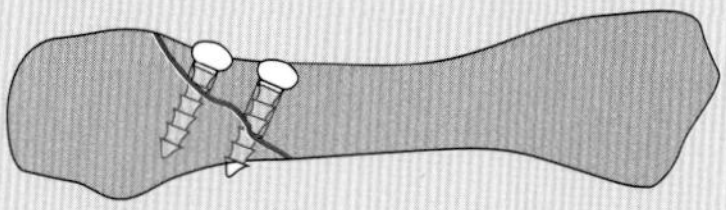	See Chapter 10.4.1, Chapter 10.6.1
	Combination of lag screw and neutralization plate 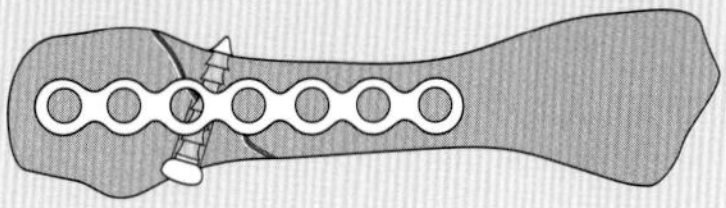	See Chapter 10.5.1

Continued ▶

Table 5.11 (*Continued*)

Fracture type	Surgical management	Procedure reference
Complex (▶ Fig. 5.30) AO: 7 1 to 5 0.3-B3 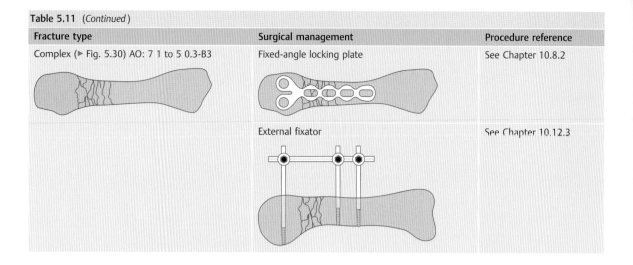	Fixed-angle locking plate	See Chapter 10.8.2
	External fixator	See Chapter 10.12.3

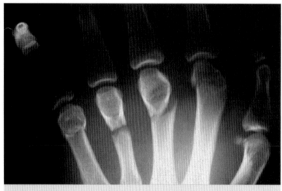

Fig. 5.28 Extra-articular metacarpal fractures, distal, transverse, left second to fifth fingers.

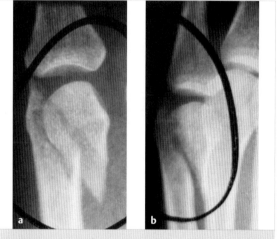

Fig. 5.29 Extra-articular metacarpal fracture, distal, spiral. X-ray in two planes (**a,b**).

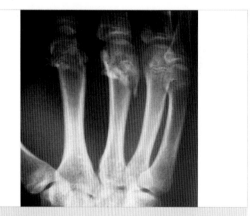

Fig. 5.30 Extra-articular metacarpal fractures, distal, complex, right second and third fingers.

5.4.3 Fractures of the Metacarpal Shaft

Table 5.12 Metacarpal shaft fractures

Fracture type	Surgical management	Procedure reference
Transverse (▶ Fig. 5.31) AO: 7 1 to 5 0.2-A1 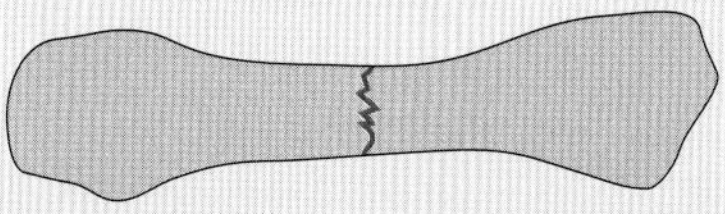	1: Wire suture, possibly with Kirschner wire	1: see Chapter 10.2.1
	2: Tension band wiring	2: see Chapter 10.3.1
	3: Compression plate (straight plate, L-, T-, H-plate)	3: see Chapter 10.7.1
	4: Fixed-angle locking plate after interfragmentary compression 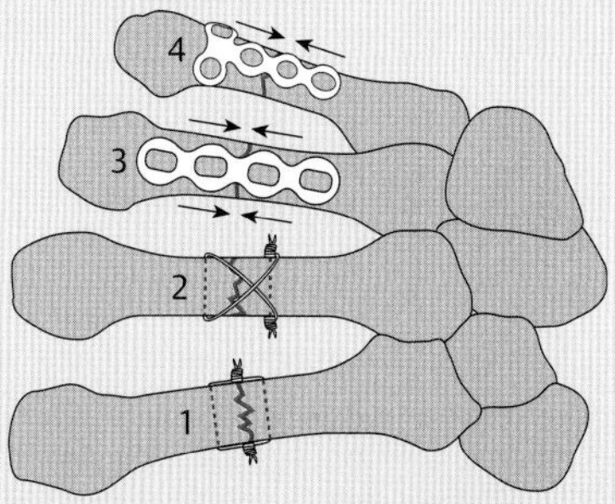	4: see Chapter 10.8.2
	Intramedullary pinning from proximal, usually open reduction 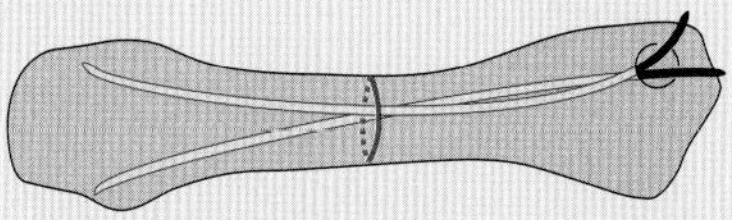	See Chapter 10.11.1
Spiral (▶ Fig. 5.32) AO: 7 1 to 5 0.2-A1 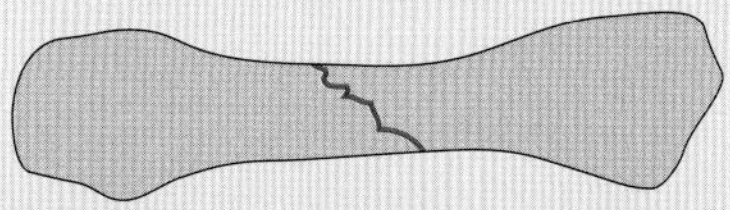	Lag screw(s) 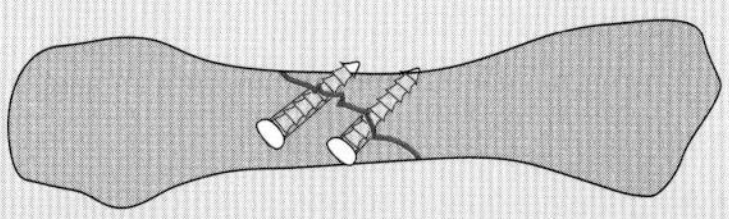	See Chapter 10.4.1, Chapter 10.6.1
	Lag screw in combination with neutralization plate 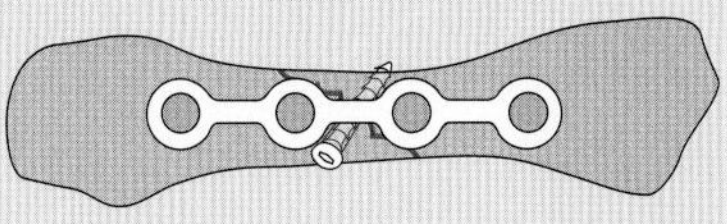	See Chapter 10.5.1
	Intramedullary pinning, usually open reduction 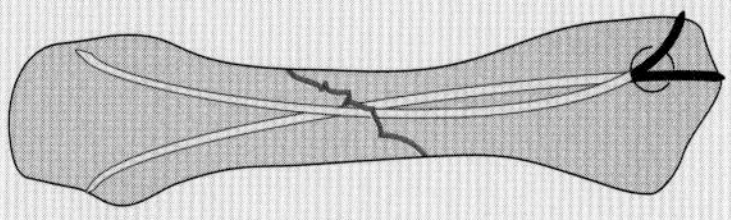	See Chapter 10.11.1
Complex AO: 7 1 to 5 0.2-A3 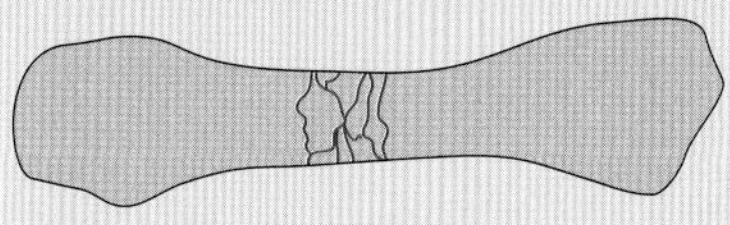	Fixed-angle locking plate 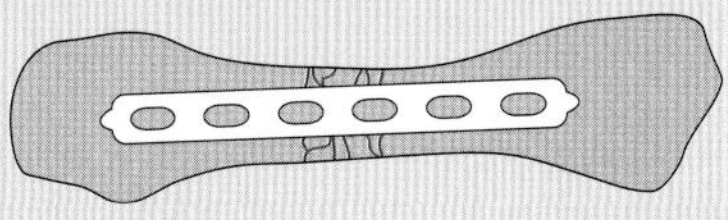	See Chapter 10.8.2
	External fixator 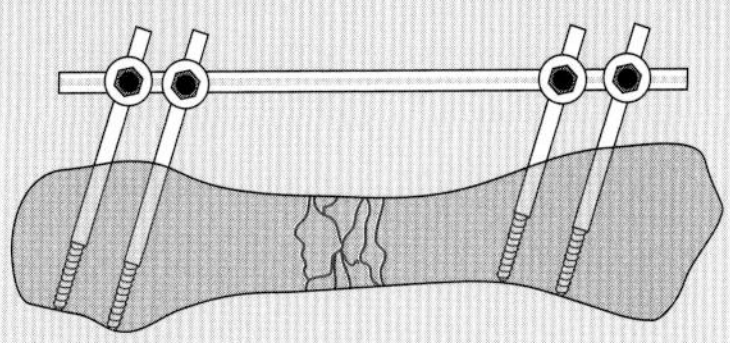	See Chapter 10.12.3

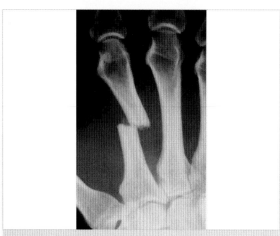

Fig. 5.31 Metacarpal shaft fracture, transverse, right second finger.

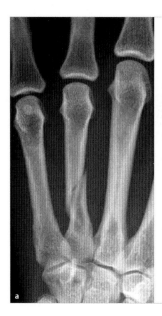
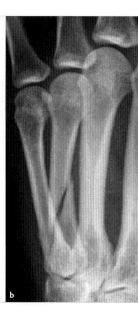

Fig. 5.32 Metacarpal shaft fracture, spiral, left fourth finger, X-ray in two planes (a,b).

5.4.4 Extra-articular Fractures of the Metacarpals, Proximal

Table 5.13 Proximal extra-articular metacarpal fractures

Fracture type	Surgical management	Procedure reference
Transverse (▶ Fig. 5.33) Spiral (▶ Fig. 5.34) AO: 7 1 to 5 0.1-B1 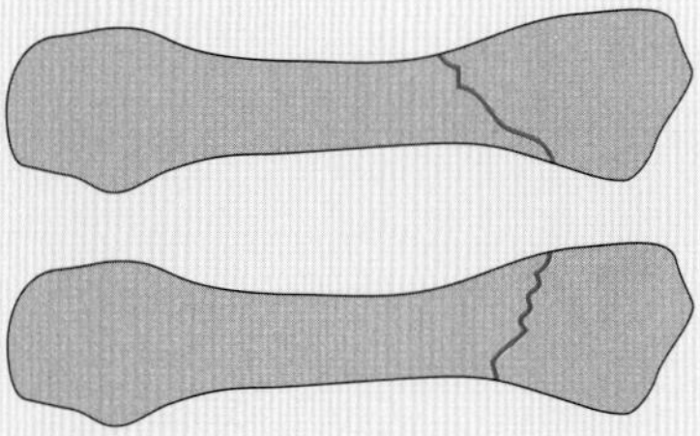	1: Percutaneous Kirschner wires 2: T-, H-plate, interfragmentary compression 3: Transfixation with Kirschner wires 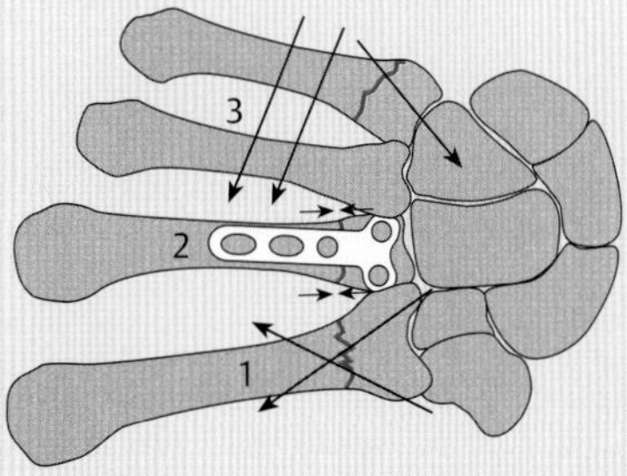	1: see Chapter 10.13.2 2: see Chapter 10.7.1 3: see Chapter 10.13.7
	Lag screw in combination with neutralization plate 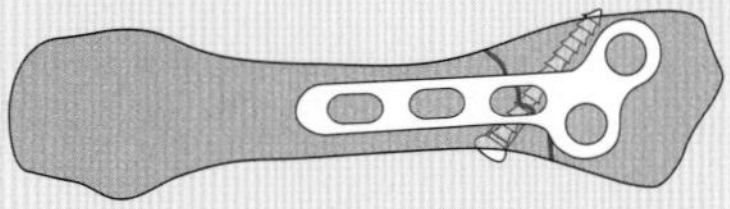	See Chapter 10.5.1
	Thumb: intramedullary pinning from distal (Kapandji) 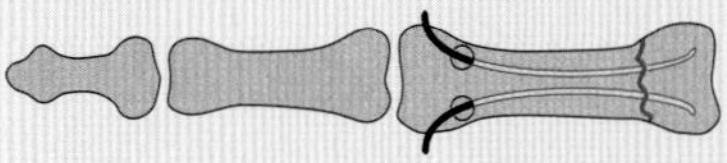	See Chapter 10.11.3
Complex AO: 7 1 to 5 0.1-B3 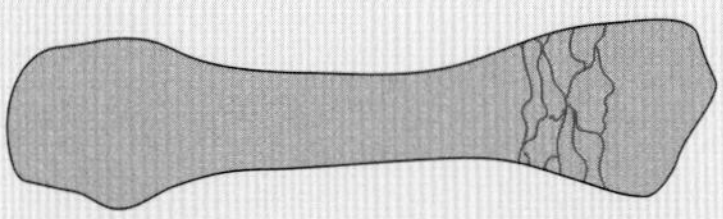	Fixed-angle locking plate 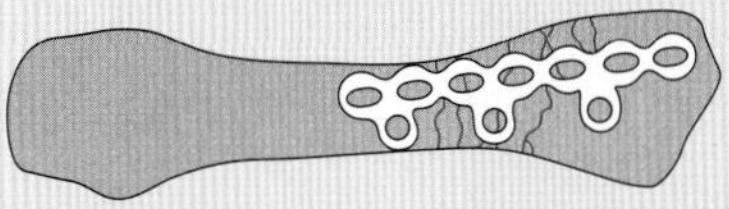	See Chapter 10.8.2

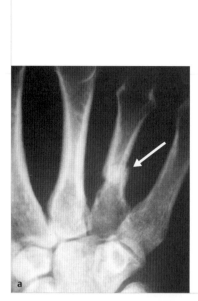

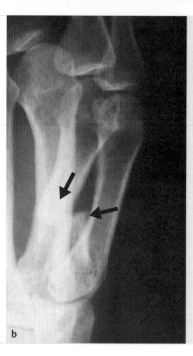

Fig. 5.33 Proximal extra-articular metacarpal fracture, transverse, right fourth finger, X-ray in two planes **(a,b)**.

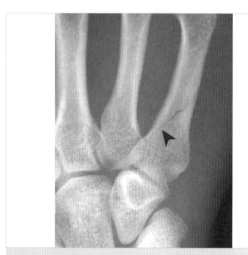

Fig. 5.34 Proximal extra-articular metacarpal fracture, spiral, right fifth finger.

5.4.5 Intra-articular Fractures of the Second to Fifth Metacarpals, Proximal

Table 5.14 Proximal intra-articular fractures of second to fifth metacarpals

Fracture type	Surgical management	Procedure reference
Border fragment (▶ Fig. 5.35) AO: 7 1 to 5 0.1-C 1	Percutaneous Kirschner wires and transfixation with Kirschner wires	See Chapter 10.13.2, Chapter 10.13.7
	Tension band wiring	See Chapter 10.3.2
	Lag screw(s), possibly with additional Kirschner wire	See Chapter 10.4.1

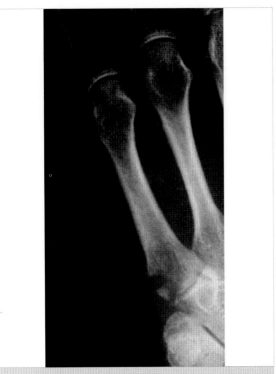

Fig. 5.35 Proximal intra-articular metacarpal fracture of left fifth finger with avulsion.

5.4.6 Intra-articular Fractures of the First Metacarpal, Proximal

Table 5.15 Intra-articular fractures of the thumb metacarpal, proximal

Fracture type	Surgical management	Procedure reference
Palmar border, Bennett fracture (▶ Fig. 5.36) AO: 7 1 0.1-C1 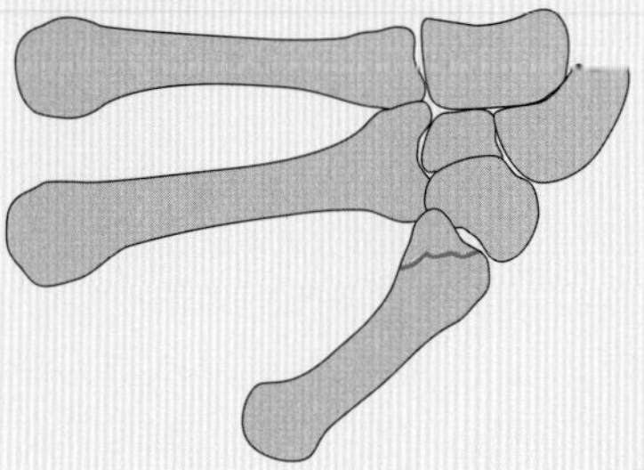	Transfixation with Kirschner wires 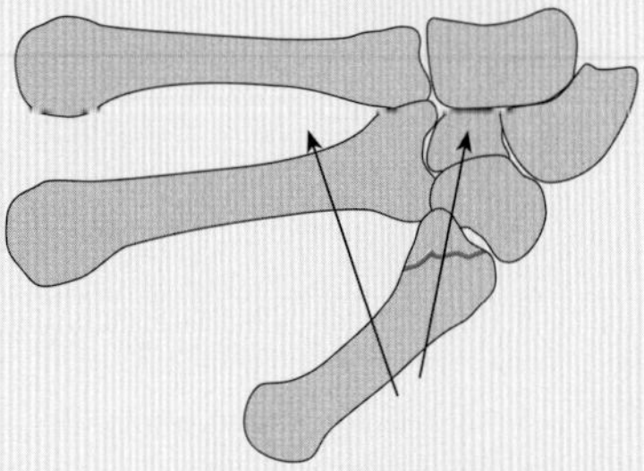 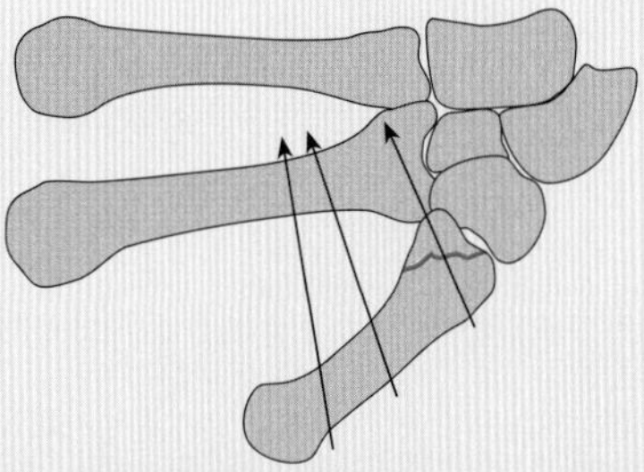	See Chapter 10.13.7
	Percutaneous Kirschner wire and/or lag screw 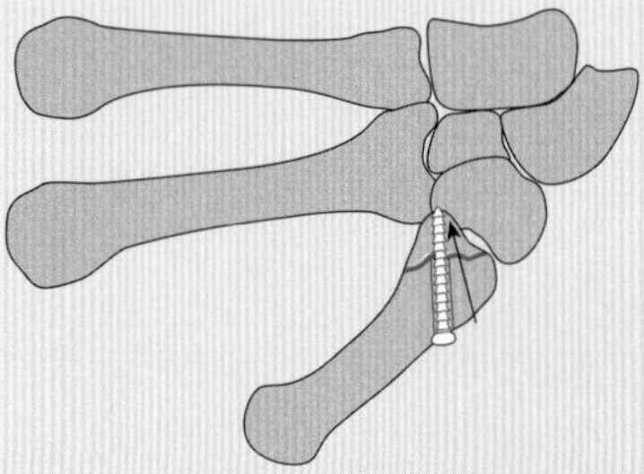	See Chapter 10.13.2, Chapter 10.4.1
	External fixator, frame construction 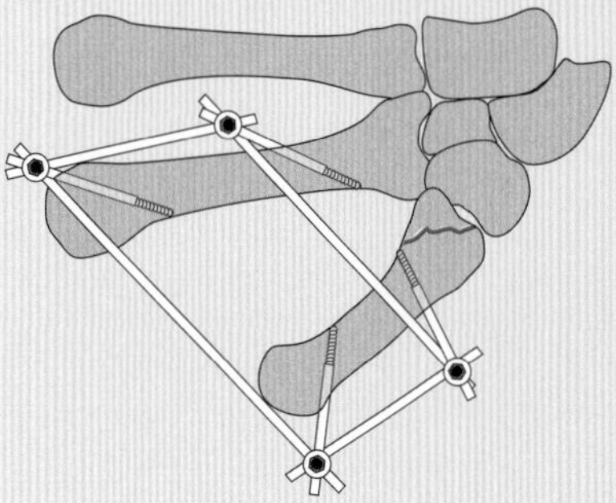	see Chapter 10.12.2, Chapter 10.12.3

Table 5.15 (*Continued*)

Fracture type	Surgical management	Procedure reference
Y, T fracture, Rolando fracture (▶ Fig. 5.37) AO: 7 1 0.1-C1 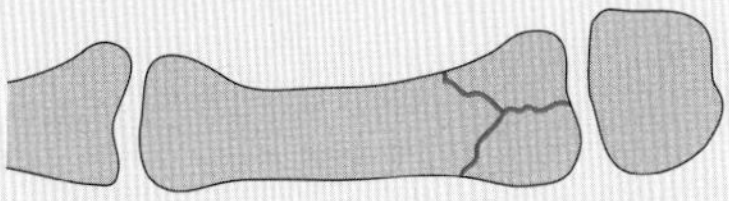 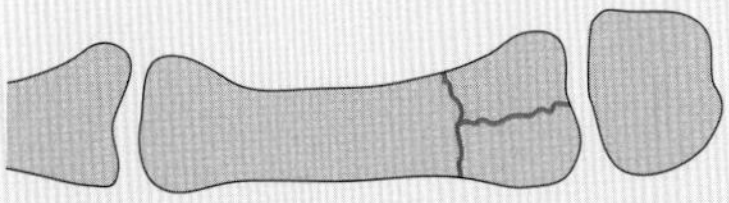	Percutaneous Kirschner wires 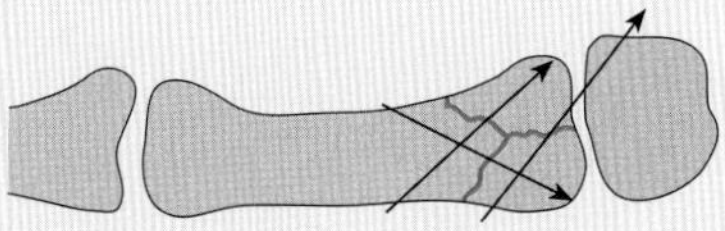	See Chapter 10.13.2
	Transfixation with Kirschner wires 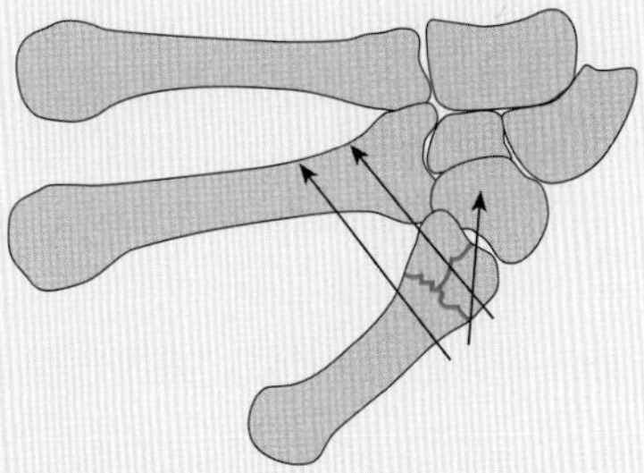	See Chapter 10.13.7
	Screw(s), with Kirschner wires 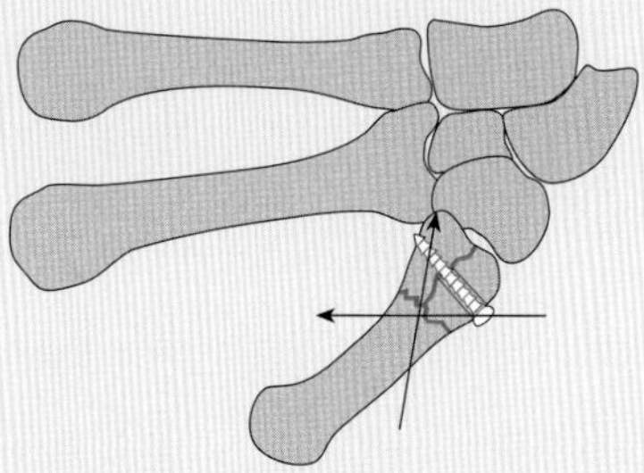	See Chapter 10.4.1
	Lag screw in combination with neutralization plate 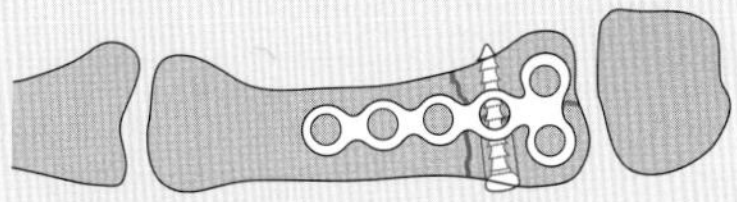	See Chapter 10.5

Continued ▶

Table 5.15 (*Continued*)

Fracture type	Surgical management	Procedure reference
Complex AO: 7 1 0.1-C3 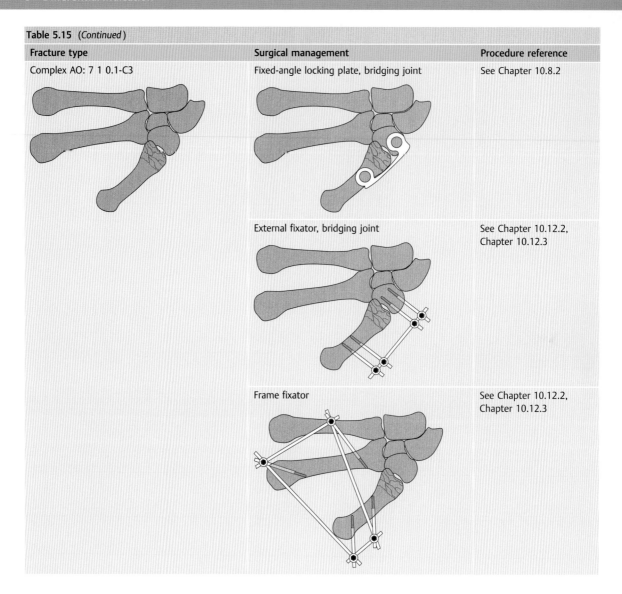	Fixed-angle locking plate, bridging joint	See Chapter 10.8.2
	External fixator, bridging joint	See Chapter 10.12.2, Chapter 10.12.3
	Frame fixator	See Chapter 10.12.2, Chapter 10.12.3

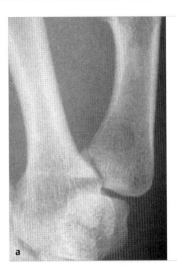
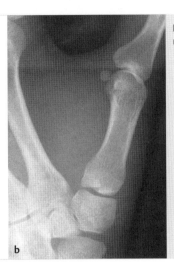

Fig. 5.36 Intra-articular fracture of base of metacarpal, right thumb: Bennett fracture (a,b).

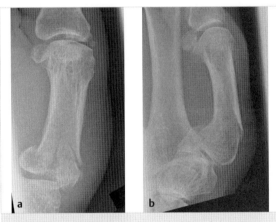

Fig. 5.37 Intra-articular T-fracture of the base of the metacarpal of the right thumb: Rolando fracture (images: Ortenau Klinikum Wolfach) (a,b).

5.5 Fractures of the Proximal Carpal Bones

5.5.1 Scaphoid Fractures

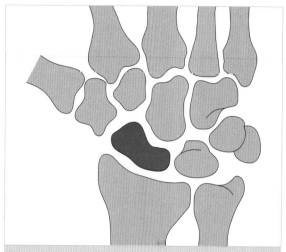

Fig. 5.38 Proximal carpal bones. The scaphoid is shown in red.

Table 5.16 Scaphoid fractures

Fracture type	Surgical management	Procedure reference
A: stable fractures, A1/A2 according to Herbert/Krimmer AO: 7 6 1.1 to 3- >A 1 to 3 • A1: tubercle (▶ Fig. 5.39a)	Cannulated lag screw	See Chapter 10.10.2

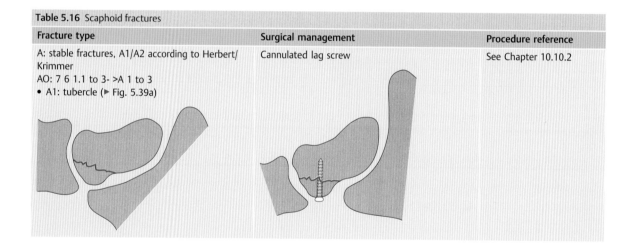

Table 5.16 (*Continued*)

Fracture type	Surgical management	Procedure reference
• A2: transverse, middle/distal third, not dislocated (▶ Fig. 5.39b) AO: 7 6 1.2–3-B 1 to 2 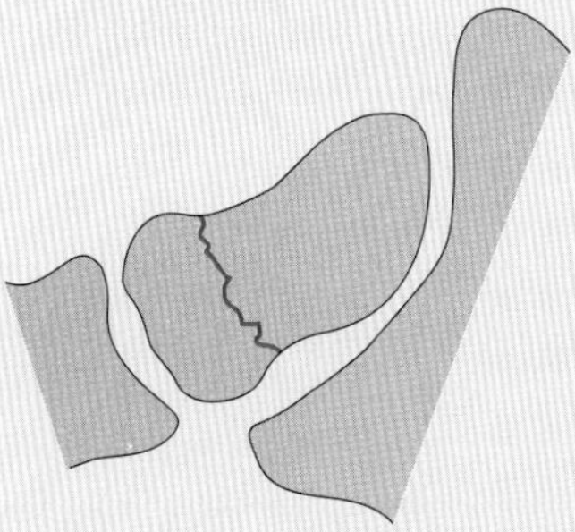	Intraosseous compression screw from distal 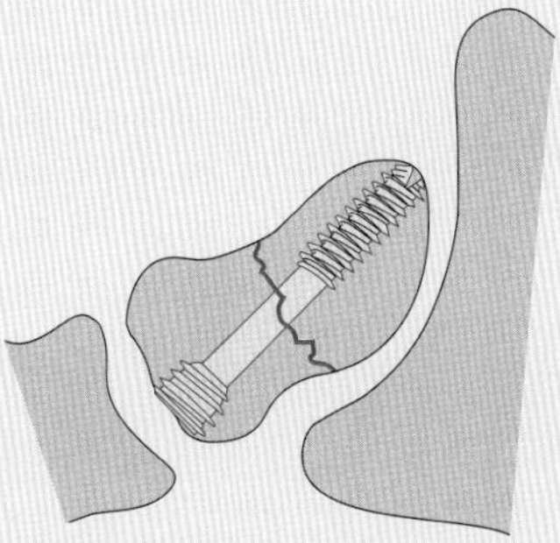	
	Cannulated lag screw plus Kirschner wire (obsolete) 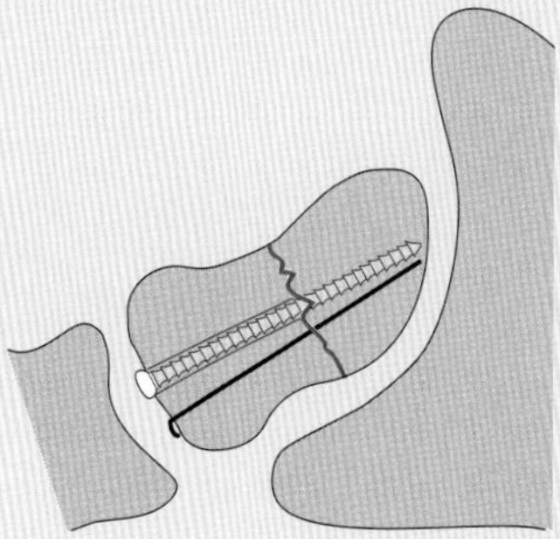	
B: unstable fractures, B1-B4 according to Herbert/ Krimmer AO: 7 6 1.1 to 3-B 1 to 3 • B1: spiral 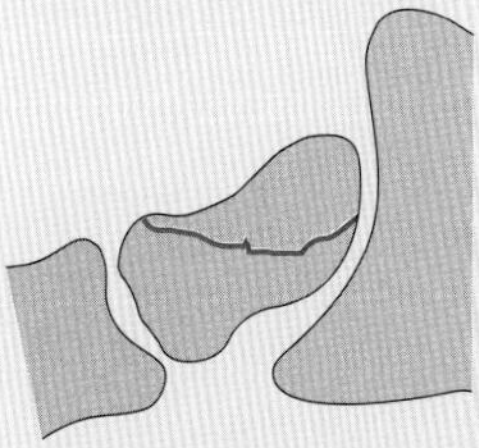	Intraosseous compression screw 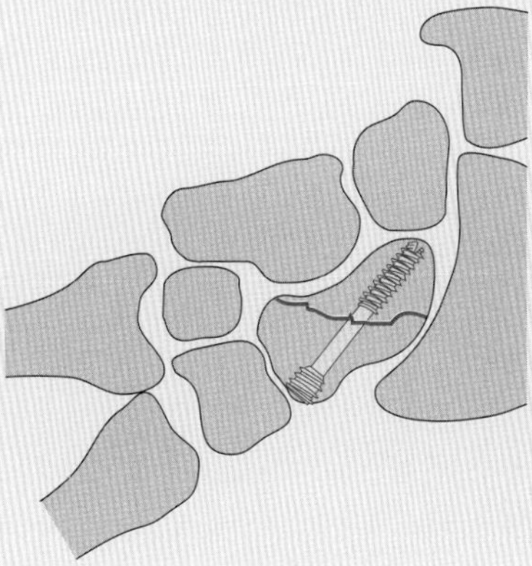	

Continued ▶

Table 5.16 (*Continued*)

Fracture type	Surgical management	Procedure reference
• B2: dislocated/gaping (► Fig. 5.40a) 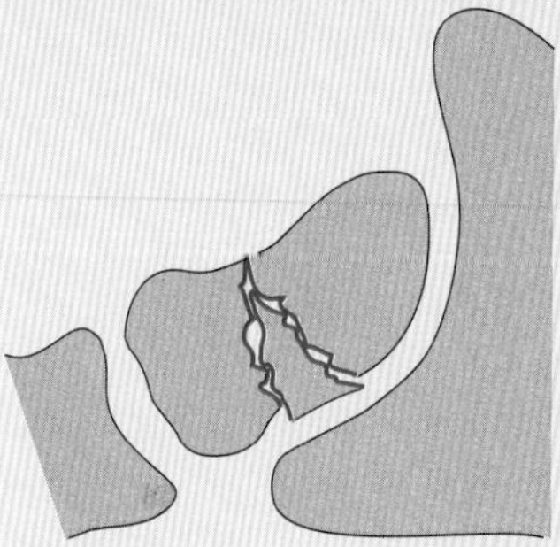 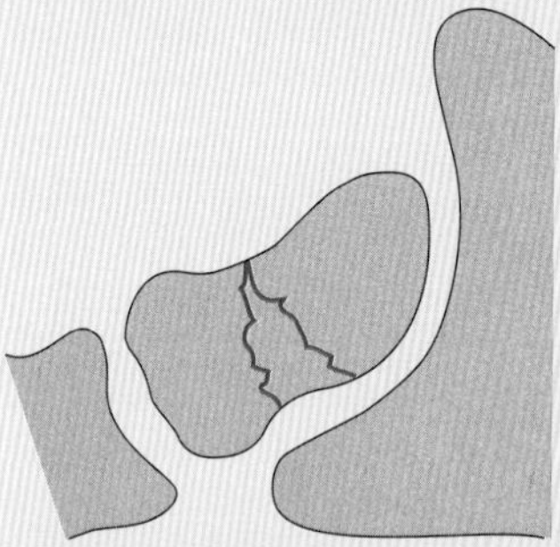	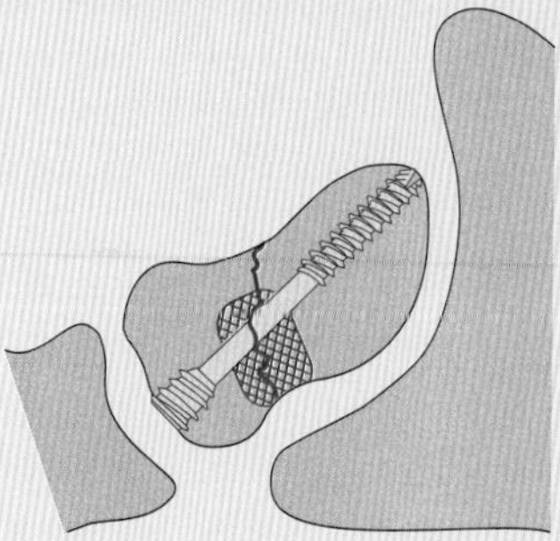 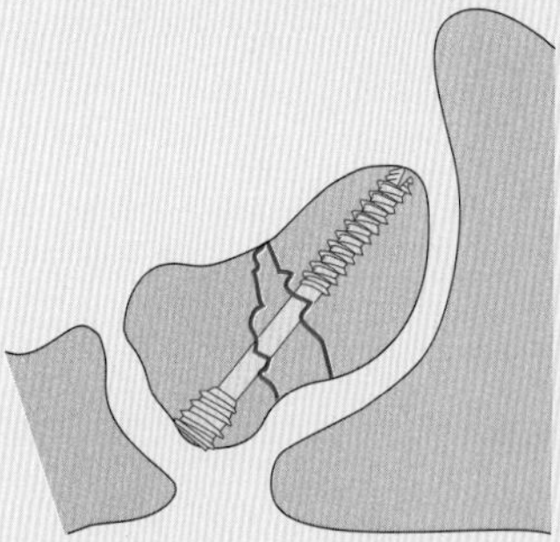	
• B3: proximal third (► Fig. 5.40b) AO: 7 6 1.3-B1 to 3 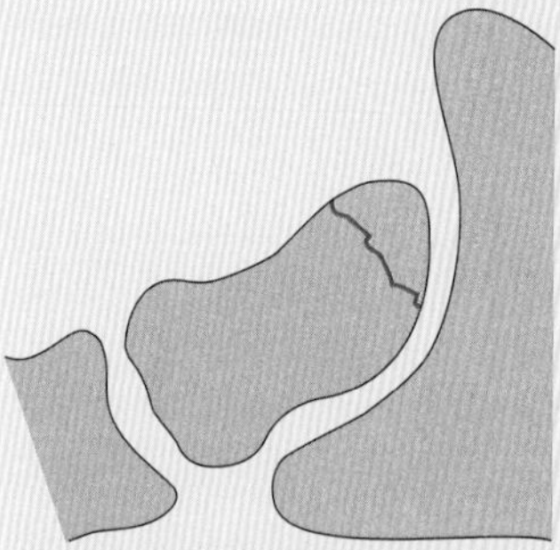	From proximal 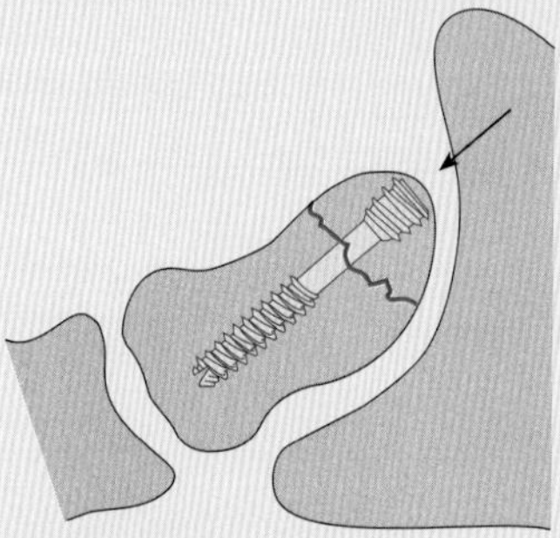	
• B4: trans-scaphoid perilunate dislocation (► Fig. 5.41)	Open reduction from palmar and/or dorsal plus internal fixation	
C: delayed union, according to Herbert/Krimmer AO: 7 6 1.1 to 3-C1 to 3 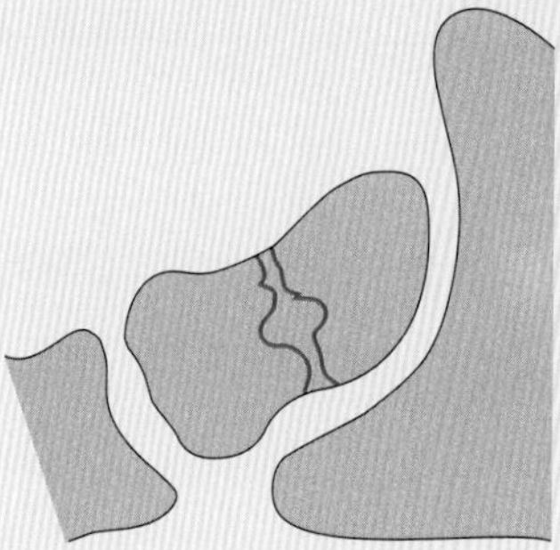	Internal fixation combined with corticocancellous bone graft 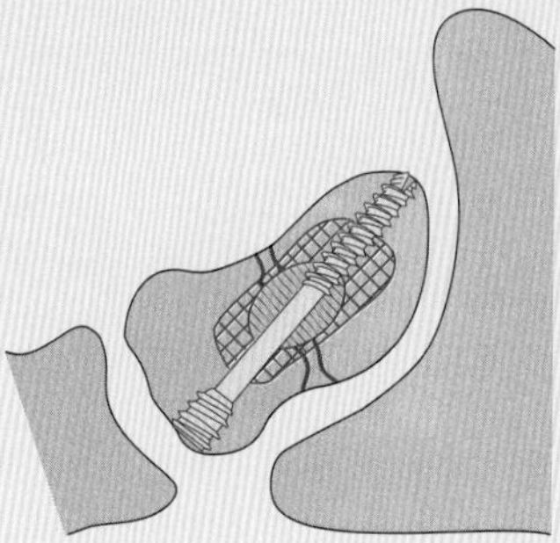	

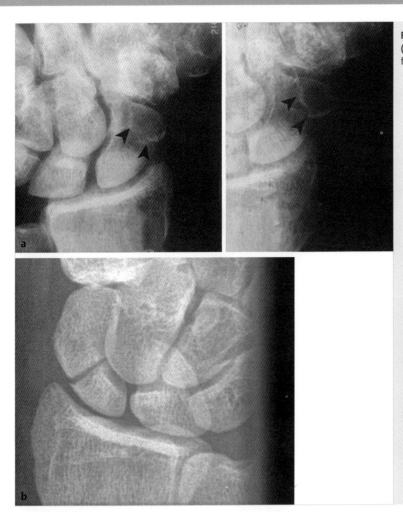

Fig. 5.39 Stable scaphoid fractures.
(a) Fracture of the tubercle. **(b)** Transverse fracture of the middle third.

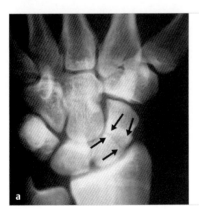 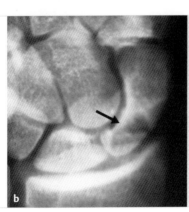

Fig. 5.40 Unstable scaphoid fractures.
(a) Transverse fracture with small wedge-shaped fragment of the radial cortex. **(b)** Fracture of the proximal third.

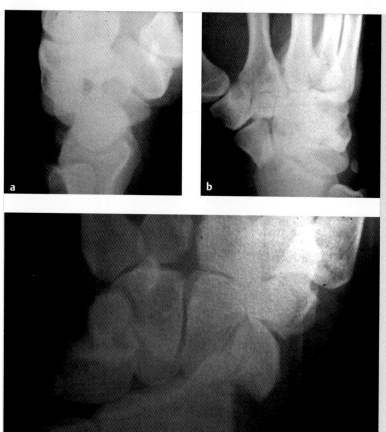

Fig. 5.41 Trans-scaphoid perilunate fracture dislocation. X-ray in three planes (a,b).

5.5.2 Lunate Fractures

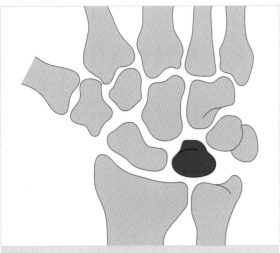

Fig. 5.42 Proximal carpal bones. The lunate is shown in red.

Table 5.17 Lunate fractures

Fracture type	Surgical management	Procedure reference
Lunate fractures (▶ Fig. 5.43) AO: 7 6 2.1 to 3-A1 to 3/B1 to 3/C1 to 3	Lag screw, possibly combined with Kirschner wire	See Chapter 10.4.1
	Intraosseous compression screw	See Chapter 10.10.2

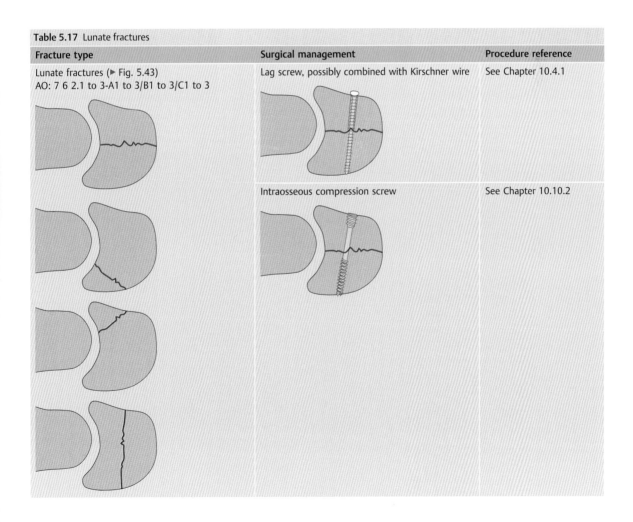

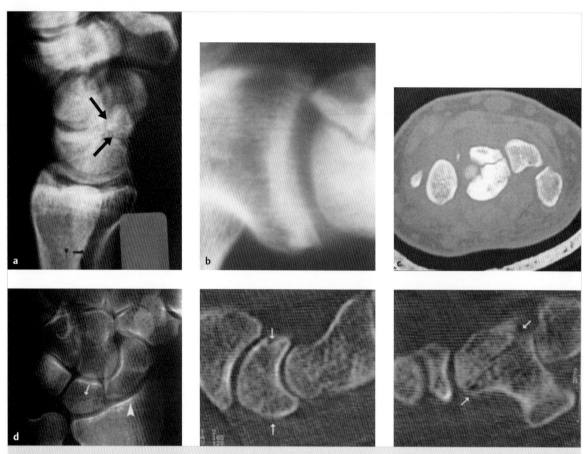

Fig. 5.43 Lunate fractures. **(a)** Shear fracture of the palmar pole: A2 fracture. **(b)** Old transverse fracture of the middle third: B2 fracture. Tomogram. **(c)** Old transverse fracture of the middle third: B2 fracture. CT scan. **(d)** Lunate fracture. Left: X-ray AP view of left wrist, combined radius fracture, radial styloid process (arrow head), lunate fracture (arrow), hamate fracture (not identifiable radiographically). Middle: CT scan, sagittal, horizontal fracture of lunate (arrows). Right: CT scan, sagittal, vertical fracture of hamate (arrows).

5.5.3 Triquetrum Fractures

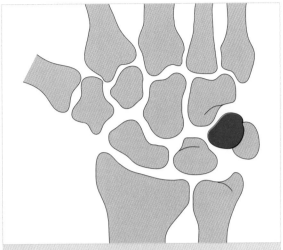

Fig. 5.44 Proximal carpal bones. The triquetrum is shown in red.

Table 5.18 Triquetrum fractures

Fracture type	Surgical management	Procedure reference
AO: 7 6 3.1 to 3-A1 to 3/B1 to 3/C1 to 3		
Chip fracture, ulnar view (▶ Fig. 5.45)	Conservative	
Simple, dorsal view (▶ Fig. 5.46)	Intraosseous compression screw	See Chapter 10.10.2
	Lag screw(s), possibly combined with Kirschner wires	See Chapter 10.4.1

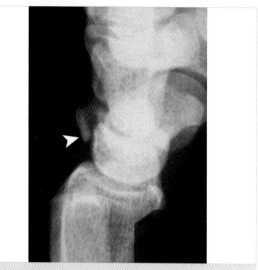

Fig. 5.45 Triquetrum fracture: dorsal shear fracture, chip fracture, A2.

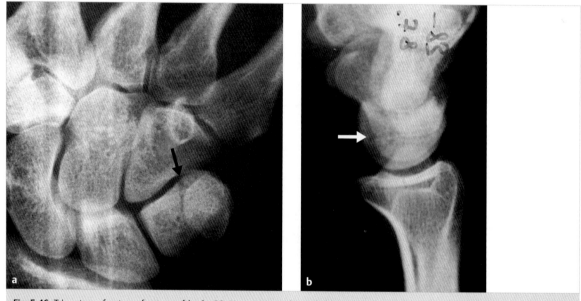

Fig. 5.46 Triquetrum fracture: fracture of body, B2. X-ray in two planes (a,b).

5.5.4 Pisiform Fractures

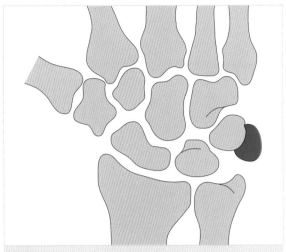

Fig. 5.47 Proximal carpal bones. The pisiform is shown in red.

Table 5.19 Pisiform fractures

Fracture type	Surgical management	Procedure reference
Simple (▶ Fig. 5.48) AO: 7 6 4.1-B1	Lag screw, intraosseous compression screw (1.7 mm—difficult)	See Chapter 10.10.2
Complex AO: 7 6 4.1-C3	Pisiform resection	

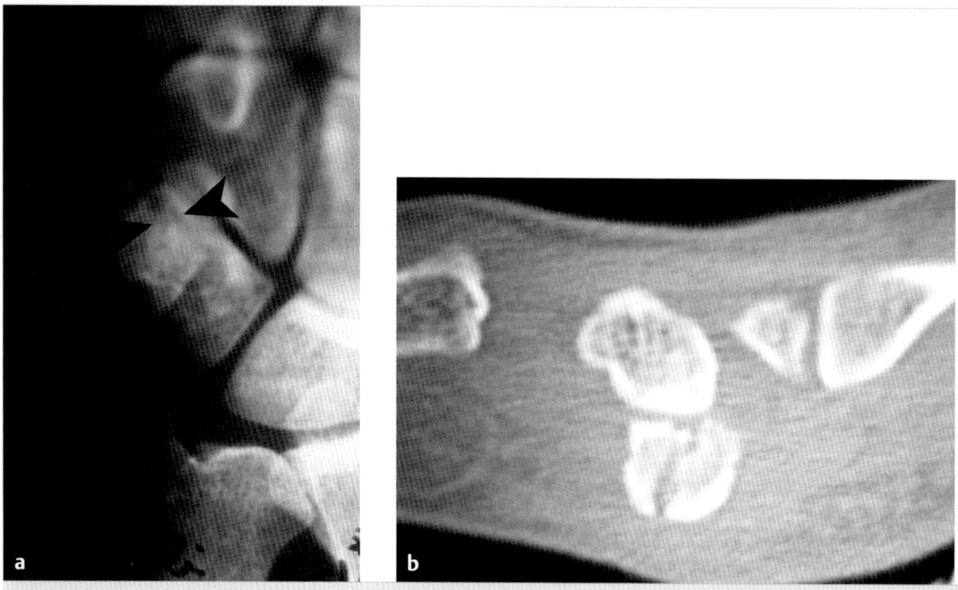

Fig. 5.48 Pisiform fracture. (a) X-ray, AP view, B3 fracture. (b) CT scan. (Image: Dr. Nägele and partners; Lahr, Schramberg.)

5.6 Fractures of the Distal Carpal Bones

5.6.1 Trapezium and Trapezoid Fractures

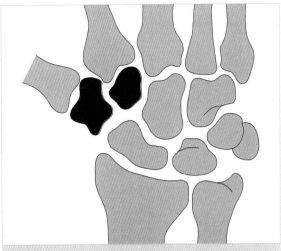

Fig. 5.49 Distal carpal bones. The trapezium and trapezoid are shown in red.

Table 5.20 Trapezium and trapezoid fractures

Fracture type	Surgical management	Procedure reference
Simple AO: 7 7 1.1 to 3-B2 and AO: 7 7 2.1 to 3-B2	Lag screw(s)	See Chapter 10.4.1

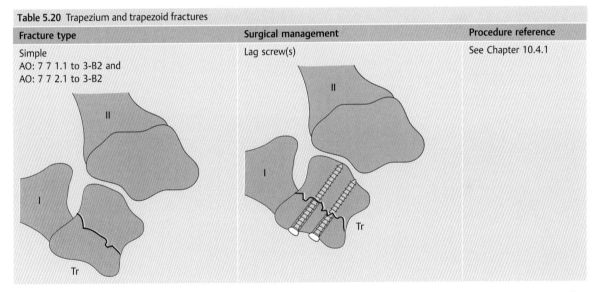

Continued ▶

Table 5.20 (Continued)

Fracture type	Surgical management	Procedure reference
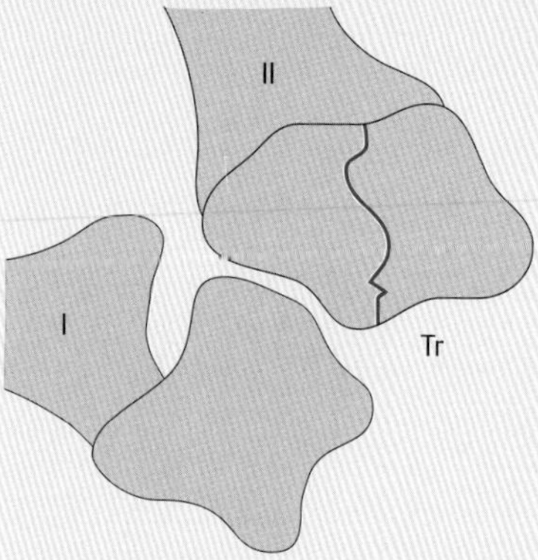	Intraosseous compression screw 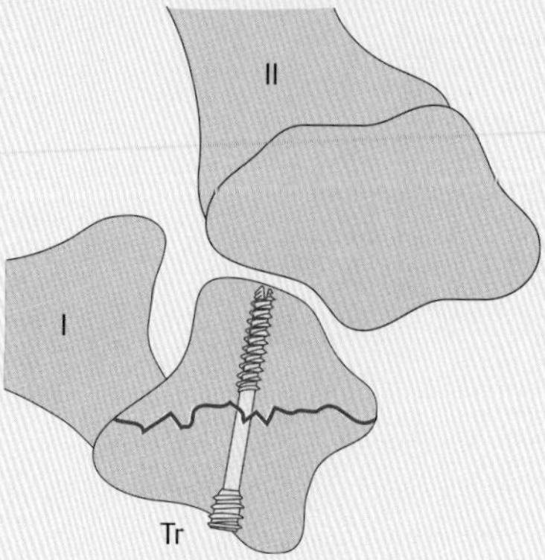	See Chapter 10.10.2
	Lag screw combined with Kirschner wire 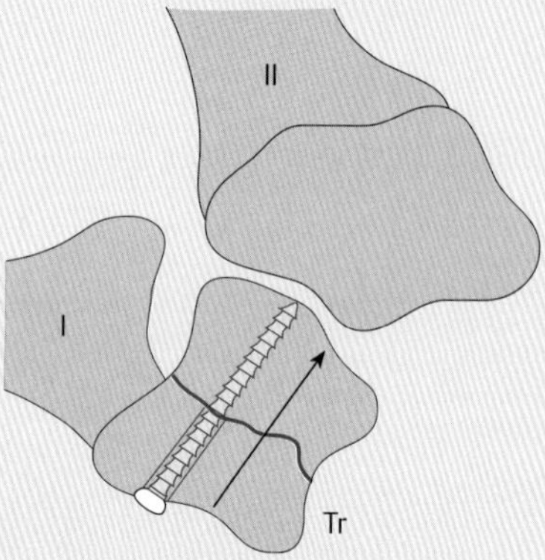 	See Chapter 10.4.1, Chapter 10.13.2
Complex AO: 7 7 1.2-C3 and AO: 7 7 2.2-C3 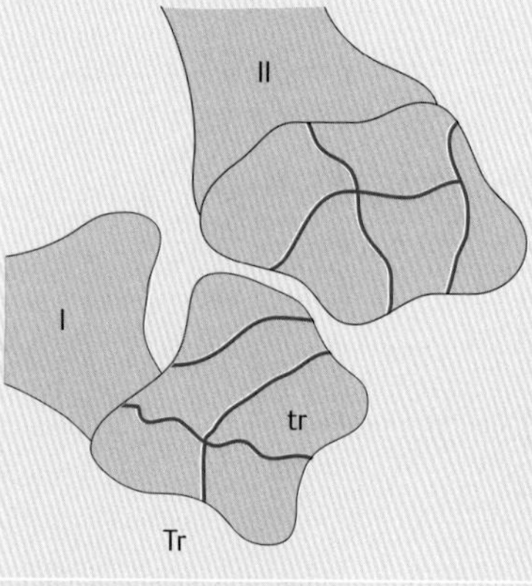 	External fixator bridging joint 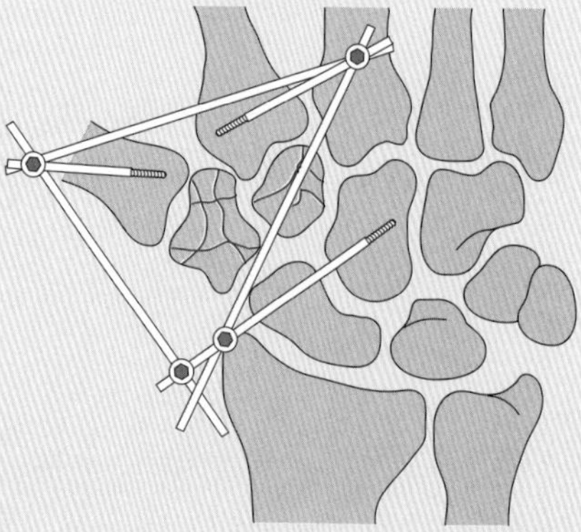 	See Chapter 10.12.2, Chapter 10.12.3

Abbreviation: Tr, trapezium.

5.6.2 Capitate Fractures

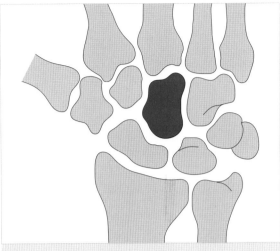

Fig. 5.50 Distal carpal bones. The capitate is shown in red.

Table 5.21 Capitate fractures

Fracture type	Surgical management	Procedure reference
AO: 7 7 3.2-B1 to 3		
Fracture of body Simple transverse (▶ Fig. 5.51) or multifragment fracture (▶ Fig. 5.52)	Transfixation with percutaneous Kirschner wires	See Chapter 10.13.7
	T-, L-, H-plate with interfragmentary compression	See Chapter 10.7.1

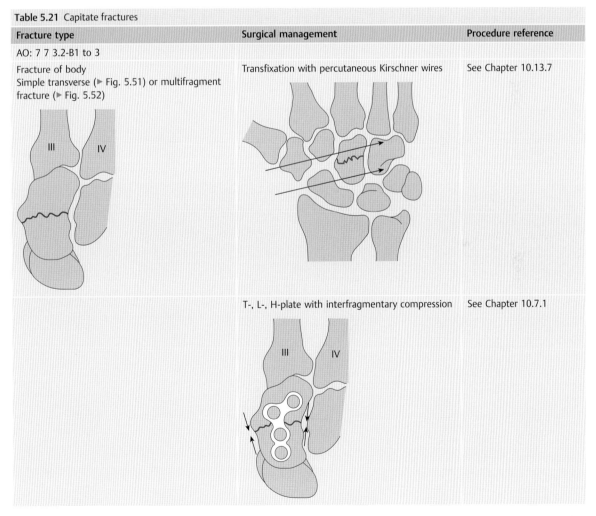

Continued ▶

Table 5.21 (*Continued*)

Fracture type	Surgical management	Procedure reference
	Intraosseous compression screw 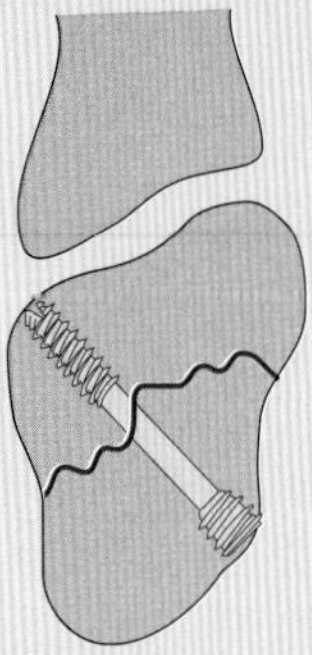 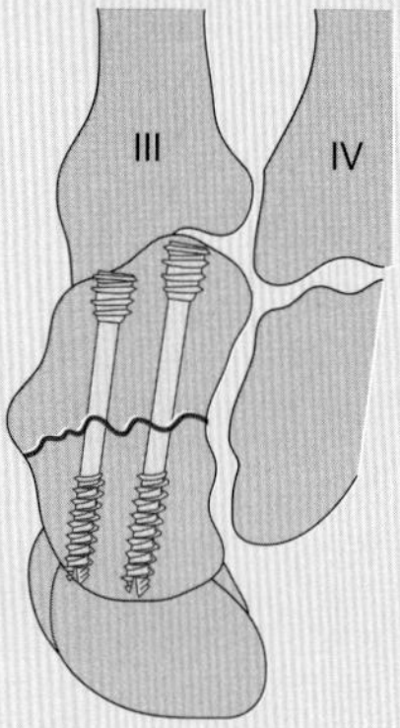	See Chapter 10.10.2
Dislocated head fragment, Fenton fracture 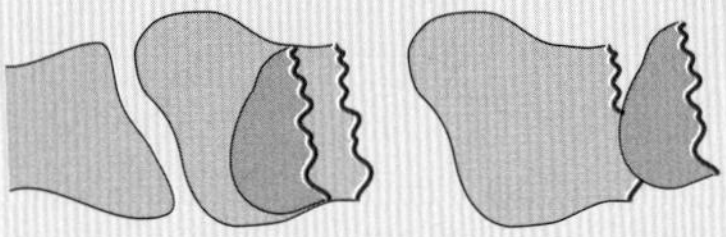	Open reduction of the fracture, then internal fixation as for transverse fracture of body	

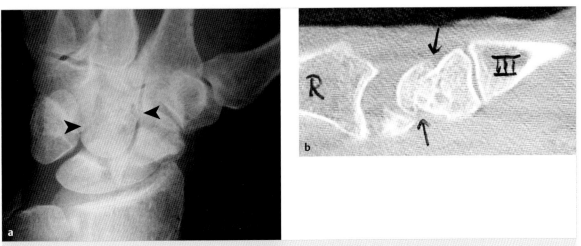

Fig. 5.51 Fracture of capitate body, transverse. **(a)** X-ray, AP view. **(b)** CT scan. (Image: Dr. Nägele and partners; Lahr, Schramberg.)

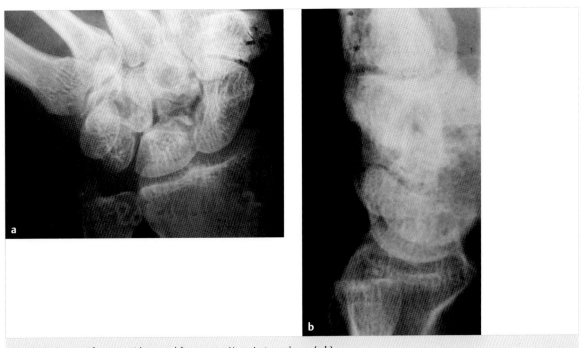

Fig. 5.52 Capitate fracture with several fragments. X-ray in two planes **(a,b)**.

5.6.3 Hamate Fractures

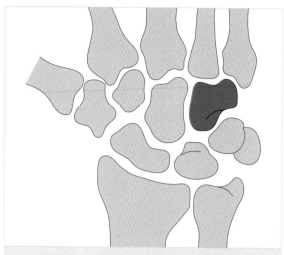

Fig. 5.53 Distal carpal bones. The hamate is shown in red.

Table 5.22 Hamate fractures

Fracture type	Surgical management	Procedure reference
AO: 7 7 4.2-B2 (A2)		
Fracture of body (dorsal view) (▶ Fig. 5.54a)	Lag screw(s) and/or percutaneous Kirschner wires	See Chapter 10.4.1, Chapter 10.13.2
Shear fracture of body (▶ Fig. 5.54b)	Lag screw(s) and/or percutaneous Kirschner wires	See Chapter 10.4.1, Chapter 10.13.2

Table 5.22 (*Continued*)

Fracture type	Surgical management	Procedure reference
Fracture of hook of hamate (ulnar view) (▶ Fig. 5.55)	Conservative Intraosseous compression screw (difficult) Resection	See Chapter 10.10.2

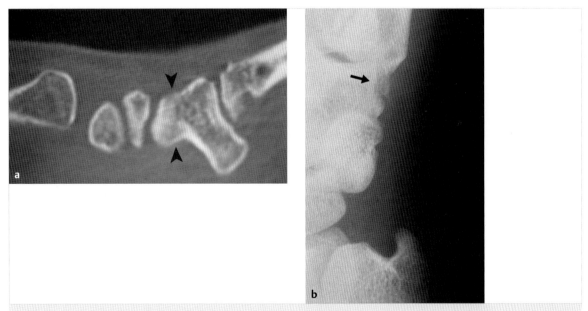

Fig. 5.54 Hamate fractures. **(a)** Fracture of body without significant dislocation, B2 fracture. (Image: Dr. Nägele and partners; Lahr, Schramberg, Germany.) **(b)** Shear fracture of the dorsal distal border of the body, A1 fracture.

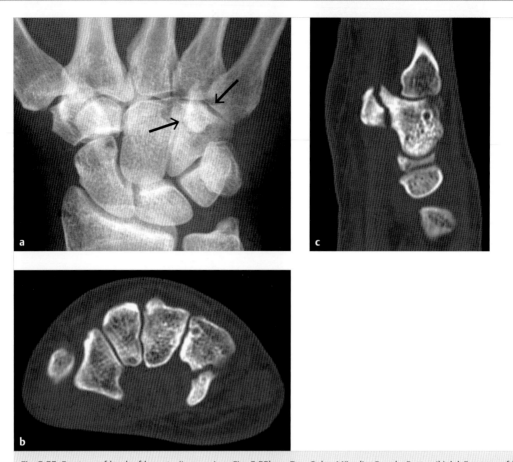

Fig. 5.55 Fracture of hook of hamate (Images in ▶ Fig. 5.55b, c: Drs. Ochs, Männlin, Rauch; Rottweil.) **(a)** Fracture of hook of hamate, slightly dislocated, A2 fracture, tennis player. **(b)** Confirmation of the fracture on CT scan, axial view. **(c)** CT, sagittal view.

Chapter 6

Principles of Surgical Management of Hand Fractures

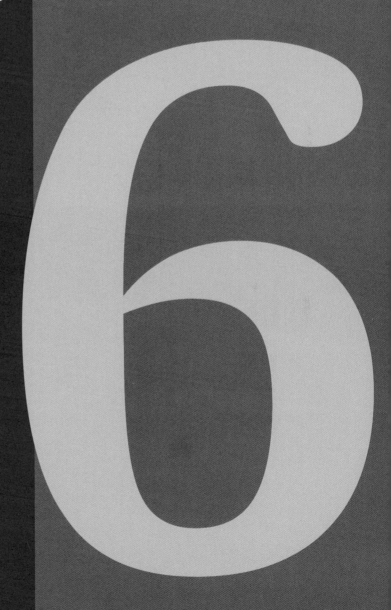

6 Principles of Surgical Management of Hand Fractures

An accurate history of the patient's injury is essential. This should include the mechanism of the accident, functional clinical examination, and precise diagnostic imaging (conventional X-ray plus CT—using high-field scanning with thin slices, if necessary and possible, and MRI). The results determine management and may decide whether or not surgery is necessary.

> **Note**
>
> The patient must always be informed of potential complications of surgical management and this information must be documented.

Hand and wrist fractures are stabilized surgically according to the following basic plan.

▶ Preoperative measures:
- Inform the patient about the extent of the injury.
- Present the treatment options: conservative or surgical; explain the advantages and disadvantages of the treatments.
- Address potential complications: impaired motion, infections, sympathetic reflex dystrophy.
- Point out the need for intensive postoperative treatment.
- Record the information provided:
  ○ General anesthesia / plexus anesthesia, complications
  ○ Screw/plate loosening
  ○ Wound infection
  ○ Absence of bony consolidation, pseudarthrosis, delayed fracture healing
  ○ Injury of sensory cutaneous nerves
  ○ Malpositioning, malalignment
  ○ Restriction of movement of uninvolved fingers
  ○ Sympathetic reflex dystrophy
  ○ Re-operation: tenolysis, repeat fixation
  ○ Postoperative arthrosis
- Precise preoperative preparation: hand bath, cleaning, drying, removal of nail varnish, sterile packing.
- Ensure that the patient is positioned comfortably on a hand table.
- Use sterile draping; if an image converter is used, do not forget to place a lead shield.
- Always apply a tourniquet cuff.

▶ Operation procedure:
- Atraumatic approach (see Chapter 9)
- Atraumatic technique ("Ten Commandments," see Chapter 4.1.1)
- Exposure of the fracture
- Meticulous anatomical reduction, as even the least imprecision leads to peripheral malalignment
- Image intensifier control
- Provisional fixation: reduction forceps, sometimes grasping fragment percutaneously, possibly temporary Kirschner wire → diameter no greater than that of screw core diameter
- Select implant size and design according to anatomical situation, fracture type, and type of injury.
- Adapt the implant: Determine plate type (standard or fixed-angle locking plate) or screw type, contour, shorten and/or bend the plate.
- Position the implant.
- Before drilling for the first hole, check rotation by flexing the fingers passively.
- Drilling: sliding hole to match screw diameter, threaded hole to match screw core diameter.
- Check that the drill bit, screw, and plate sizes do match.
- Whenever possible, obtain interfragmentary compression: lag screw(s), dynamic fixation, compression by means of reduction forceps.
- Maintain reduction and stability by final fixation.
- Establish and document whether the internal fixation is rigid, loading-stable or limited, and motion-stable.
- Final hemostasis by bipolar cautery
- Atraumatic wound closure without tension, preferably without a drain
- Intraoperative/postoperative X-ray
- Sterile dressing, if necessary applying a splint for immobilization
- Elevation of the arm

▶ Postoperative measures:
- Explain further treatment to the patient in detail
- Postoperative early functional treatment: physical therapy, ergotherapy

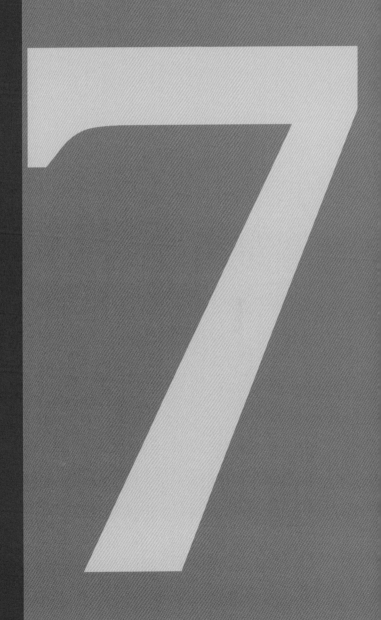

Chapter 7

Postoperative Treatment

7 Postoperative Treatment

No matter how accurate the internal fixation, a successful outcome largely depends on the postoperative treatment. After surgery, edema is caused by accumulation of excessive fluid in the intercellular space. This swelling diminishes perfusion and may lead to congestion, *dysregulation*, and increased risk of infection. Pain and immobilization result in muscle atrophy. Muscle and ligament contractures decrease the range of motion. The following postoperative measures are essential:

▶ **Analgesia and exercise therapy.** Adequate analgesia must be ensured as otherwise the patient will likely not tolerate or actively participate in appropriate postoperative treatment. Priority should be given to an effective and more consistent application of preferably active mobilization, muscle pump activity by active isometric muscle exercise, wherever possible, and elevation of the limb above shoulder height. Instructions must be repeated often and emphatically! Slings should be avoided.

▶ **Wound monitoring.** Regular dressing changes, under analgesia/anesthesia (children) if necessary, are essential. The plaster cast should be checked for cleanliness, fit, functional position, and pressure sites, and replaced if necessary. Hematomas must be evacuated surgically under sterile conditions. Partially opening the wound or removing sutures is not sufficient in this case.

▶ **Early mobilization.** Early mobilization starts as soon as possible, depending on the wound and the patient's general condition. Physical therapy for the shoulder and elbow starts on the first postoperative day to avoid disorders in the chain of movements of the upper extremity. Proprioceptive neuromuscular facilitation (PNF) techniques are helpful.

Depending on progress, mobilization is increased with controlled physical therapy, which is supplemented by occupational therapy later on. Independent activity by the patient is encouraged. Active physical therapy is preferable to passive measures.

▶ **Additional measures.** Additional physical measures include intermittent ice application for pain relief and to improve perfusion.

When used appropriately, passive exercises can help to prevent adhesions of tendons and sliding surfaces. Treatment can be supported by manual therapy to maintain rolling and sliding joint movements with traction and translation.

Lymph drainage reduces swelling but is only indicated after the wound is well healed.

Treatment of scars consisting of pressure dressings, compression hose, and compression gloves is occasionally helpful. After complete wound healing, scar ointments will have a positive effect, not least for psychological reasons.

▶ **Occupational therapy.** As soon as the internal fixation is stable on motion and loading, physical therapy must be supplemented with occupational therapy. Functional improvements are achieved by having the patient perform active tasks with the injured hand in order to attain pain-free precision, power, and key grips. The occupational therapy repertoire also includes **self-help** training, provision of aids and, if necessary, use of a dynamic splint. Sensibility training to improve sensation should not be neglected.

> **Note**
>
> The importance of physical therapy and occupational therapy must be emphasized. Optimal internal fixation is worth little without them.
>
> The quality of hand therapy must be ensured, however. Preference should be given to therapists with a certified qualification in hand therapy, as provided by specialist courses.

Chapter 8

Implants and Instruments

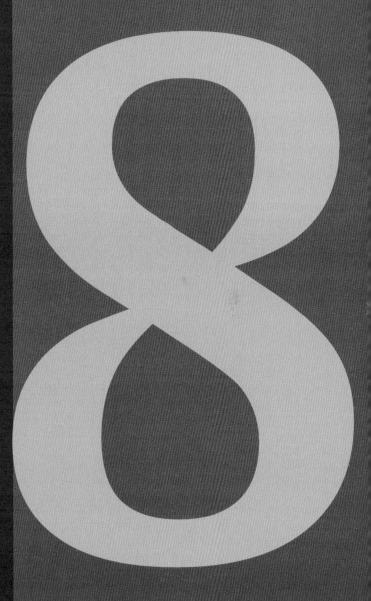

8 Implants and Instruments

8.1 General Remarks

Significant technical improvements to implants and instruments have been achieved. The dimensions and designs have been adapted to the anatomy of the hand.

They have slender profiles and can be used for different bone shapes and fracture types. The rounded edges cause minimal trauma. With the introduction of titanium, allergenic components have largely disappeared.

Self-tapping screws in all sizes are the norm today. Thread-tapping instruments are a thing of the past.

8.2 Fixed-Angle Locking Fixation

> **Note**
>
> The development of fixed-angle locking fixation has contributed greatly to the safety of postoperative loading.

This requires a stable connection between screw and plate. Different options are provided by the industry:
- Unidirectional fixed-angle locking fixation
- Multidirectional fixed-angle rigid fixation by means of locking

▶ **Unidirectional connection.** The thread of the screw head and the thread of the plate hole are identical. Tightening the screw in the hole produces a firm connection between screw and plate. With this kind of connection, the direction of the screw and plate is predetermined; it therefore is called a unidirectional connection (▶ Fig. 8.1).
▶ **Multidirectional connection by means of locking.** Locking is based on two different technical methods, both of which lead to a stable connection through plastic deformation of the thread of the screw and the plate hole. One method locks the thread of the screw head in the plate hole through a reshaping process due to differences in material hardness and design. The other method uses a jamming mechanism between one lip of the plate and the head-thread of the screw while locking (▶ Fig. 8.2). The multidirectional locking method allows variance when placing the fixed-angle locking screws up to an angle of 20° between screw and plate (▶ Fig. 8.3).

▶ **Advantages and disadvantages.** Fixed-angle locking fixation allows the components to become ever smaller in size, which is naturally an advantage given the delicacy of the hand and finger structures. Nevertheless, fixed-angle locking plates are thicker than standard implants.

Because fixed-angle fixation is rigid, implant placement outside the tension band side is possible. Sensitive gliding

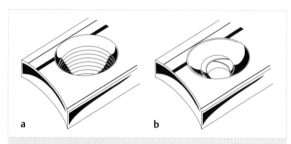

Fig. 8.2 Fixed-angle locking plate holes. **(a)** Unidirectional with precisely defined thread. **(b)** Multidirectional, threaded lip for locking.

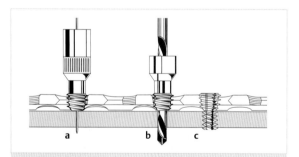

Fig. 8.1 Methodical placement of unidirectional fixed-angle locking screws. **(a)** The unidirectional drill guide is fixed in the plate. **(b)** The hole is drilled with the diameter of the screw core. **(c)** The fixed-angle locking screw is tightened until the screw head is countersunk in the plate.

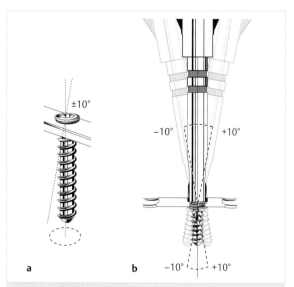

Fig. 8.3 (a,b) Conical variant for placing multidirectional fixed-angle locking screws.

structures, especially the extensor tendons, are less traumatized, thereby minimizing the feared adhesions.

A further advantage is preservation of periosteal perfusion, as the stability of the fixation is based on the principle of rigid internal fixator stability and not on friction between the plate and the bone surface (▶ Fig. 8.4).

All of these factors contribute to a more secure fracture healing and, when used correctly, reduce the typical complications of surgically treated fractures.

The disadvantage is the higher financial *cost* compared with conventional standard implants.

8.3 Screws

Screws with diameters of 1.0, 1.2, 1.3, 1.5, 1.6, 1.7, 2.0, 2.3, and 2.4 mm are now available depending on the manufacturer (▶ Fig. 8.5). Fixed-angle locking screws come with diameters of 1.4, 1.5, 1.7, 2.0, 2.3, and 2.4 mm (▶ Fig. 8.6).

The driving recess of screw heads and screwdriver bits have different designs, ranging from cross-head, square, and hexagonal to star-shaped (▶ Fig. 8.7).

Precise documentation of the materials used is essential so that the corresponding instruments are available if implant removal becomes necessary.

The design dimensions are denoted by letters (XS, S, M, L, Mini, Midi) and may also be color coded so that corresponding screws and plates can be coordinated readily.

Knowledge of the screw diameter and the screw core diameter is necessary as this determines the size of the hole to be predrilled for a fixation screw or lag screw (▶ Fig. 8.8).

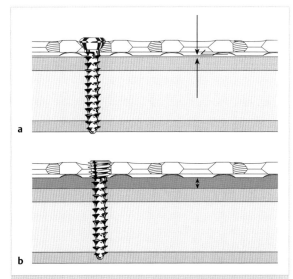

Fig. 8.4 The stability of plate fixation is based on two different principles. **(a)** Friction principle: Stability is achieved by friction between the plate and the bone surface. **(b)** Fixed-angle locking principle: This corresponds to an internal fixator; that is, stability is achieved by a rigid construction between plate and screw. An advantage is that perfusion of the periosteum is not affected because of the gap between plate and bone surface.

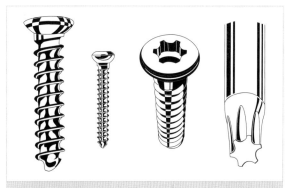

Fig. 8.5 Standard cortical screws.

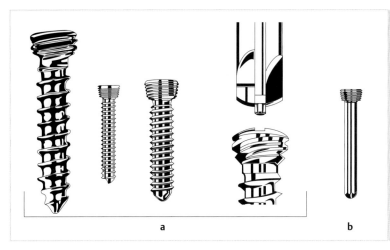

Fig. 8.6 Fixed-angle locking screws. **(a)** Unidirectional and multidirectional fixed-angle screws. **(b)** Fixed-angle pin.

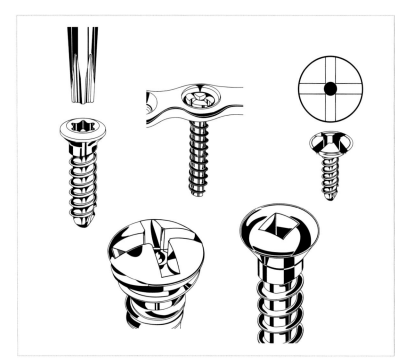

Fig. 8.7 Different designs of screw-head driving recess.

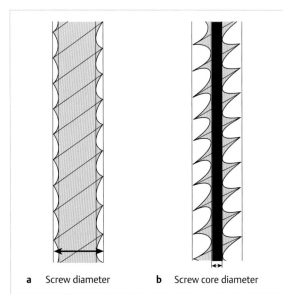

a Screw diameter   **b** Screw core diameter

Fig. 8.8 Screw and screw core diameter. **(a)** When a gliding hole is drilled, the diameter matches the diameter of the screw. **(b)** When a fixation hole is drilled, the diameter of the pilot hole must correspond to the diameter of the screw core.

8.4 Plates

The dimensions of the plates must fit the anatomy. The variety of designs and dimensions is almost unlimited. It is important to make sure that screw and plate match (color coding). Plate designs come in different sizes and models (▶ Fig. 8.9):

- Straight plates, adaptation plates, locking compression plates (LCP), etc.
- T-plates
- L-plates
- H-plates
- Y-plates
- Z-plates
- Condylar plates
- Strut plates
- 3-D plates
- Grid plates
- Trapezoid plates
- Mesh modules
- Double plates
- Rotation plates

The profile height of standard plates is lower than that of fixed-angle plates, which is between 0.6 and 1.5 mm.

▶ **Plate holes.** The plate holes are guided by plate function (▶ Fig. 8.10):

- Combined hole
- Locking hole
- Oval hole
- Round hole
- Adaptation hole

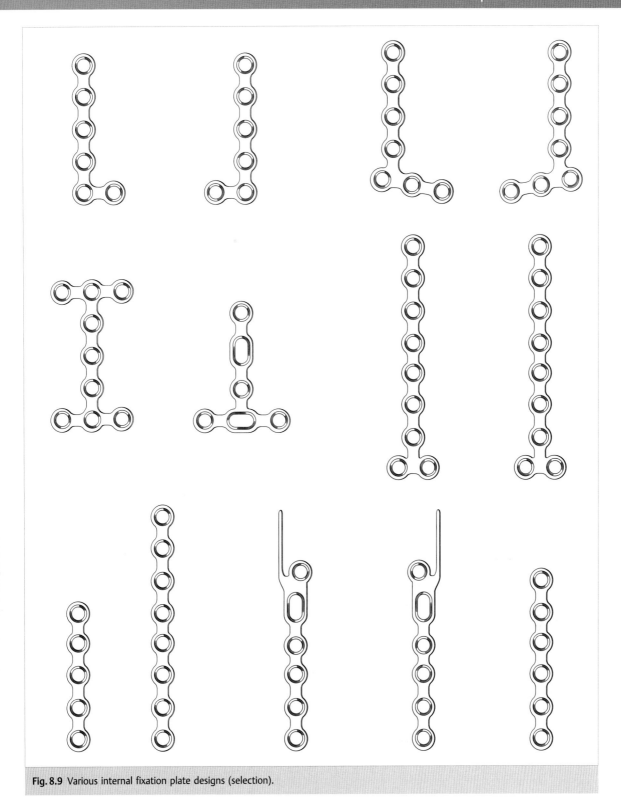

Fig. 8.9 Various internal fixation plate designs (selection).

Continued ▶

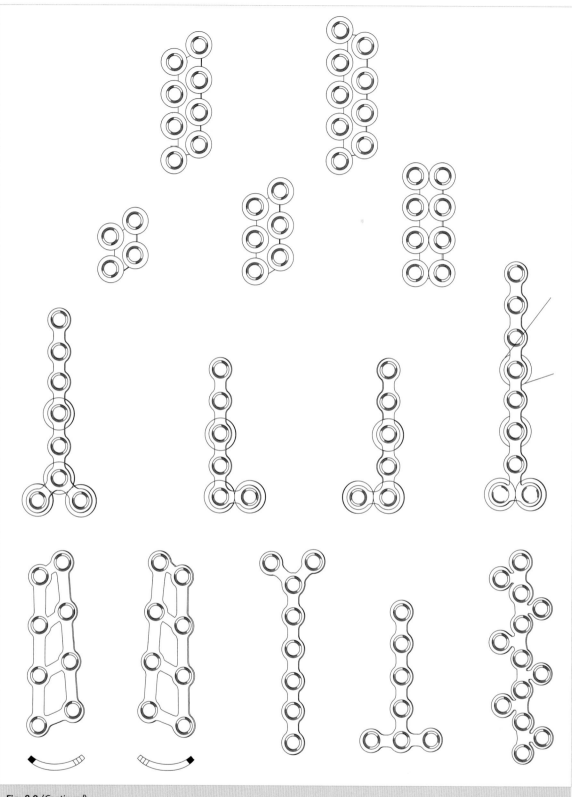

Fig. 8.9 (*Continued*)

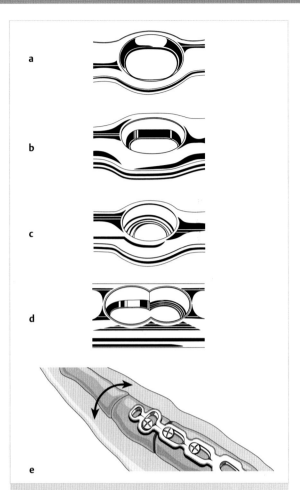

Fig. 8.10 Varieties of plate holes. **(a)** Compression hole. **(b)** Oval compression hole. Compression holes and oval compression holes are suitable exclusively for standard cortical screws. With noneccentric drilling, fixation is by friction; with asymmetrical drilling, displacement of the plate relative to the bone can be achieved through the gliding hole principle. **(c)** Locking hole suitable for standard cortical screws→ stability by friction; also suitable for fixed-angle screws: screw and plate—internal fixator. **(d)** Combined hole, suitable both for standard cortical screws and for fixed-angle screws. **(e)** Rotation hole allows correction of rotation error when a plate is already fixed in a fragment.

Chapter 9

Surgical Approaches

9 Surgical Approaches

9.1 General Remarks

To avoid risks and complications due to incisions, these should be made on the flexor side of the hand or finger, usually in a zigzag (Bruner) but sometimes in an **L** or **S** shape. By contrast, straight incisions are possible on the extensor aspect of the hand; however, these should pass laterally to the joints. Straight incisions should not be made directly over the extensor tendons, so as to avoid adhesions due to scarring.

Scars on the sensitive fingertips and edges of the hand interfere with hand function. Whenever possible, the radial side of the index, middle and ring fingertips and the ulnar side of the little fingertip should be spared.

Structures that run longitudinally, nerves, and vessels must be noted particularly. Veins that run longitudinally must be preserved, whereas transversely running veins may be ligated if necessary.

If deeper structures have to be divided to obtain adequate vision, they must be divided in a way that they can be repaired by suture. This applies particularly to extensor tendons, ligaments, and joint capsule.

> **Note**
>
> Scars in the region of tendon sutures and internal fixation material tend to form considerable adhesions, which in turn leads to major delay in restoration of function due to scar retraction.

9.2 Palmar Approach to the Distal Phalanx, Distal Interphalangeal Joint, and Distal Middle Phalanx

- Incise the skin in zigzag fashion according to Bruner (▶ Fig. 9.1a).
- Expose and incise laterally the A5 annular pulley and C3 cruciate pulley to expose the insertion of the deep flexor tendon (▶ Fig. 9.1b).

> **Practical Tip**
>
> Preserve the vessels and nerves on the radial and ulnar sides and, if possible, the A4 annular pulley.

- Reflect the divided annular pulleys laterally; retract the distal deep flexor tendon with a blunt retractor to expose the palmar plate (▶ Fig. 9.1c).
- To obtain access to the joint, divide the palmar plate gradually as far as needed (▶ Fig. 9.1c).

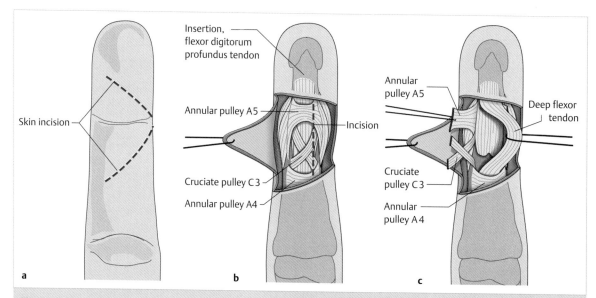

Fig. 9.1 Palmar approach to the proximal distal phalanx, distal interphalangeal joint, and distal middle phalanx. **(a)** Skin incision. **(b)** The skin and subcutaneous tissue are elevated together from the extensor sheath and retracted with retaining sutures. The radial/ulnar neurovascular bundles (not shown) are protected and the tendon sheath is incised laterally. **(c)** Retaining sutures are placed in the divided A5 pulley, the deep flexor tendon is retracted laterally, and the palmar plate is exposed.

9.3 Dorsal Approach to the Distal Phalanx, Distal Interphalangeal Joint, and Distal Middle Phalanx

- Perform the skin incision over the dorsal joint crease, preferably in **Y**, **H**, or **S** shape (▶ Fig. 9.2a).
- Retract the skin flaps by fine retaining sutures and expose the insertion of the extensor tendon on the distal phalanx (▶ Fig. 9.2b).

- Expose the distal interphalangeal joint by oblique / lazy S-shaped division of the distal extensor tendon (▶ Fig. 9.2c).

Caution

Protect the nail matrix to avoid deformity of the nail.

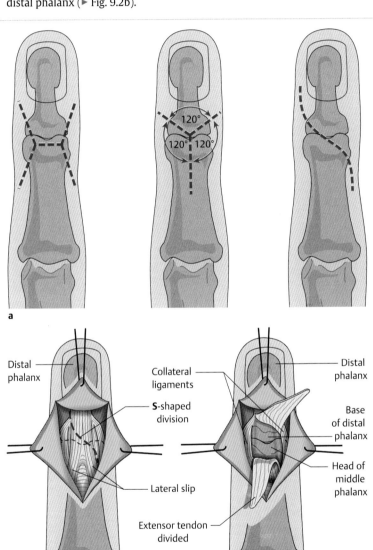

Distal phalanx

Collateral ligaments

S-shaped division

Lateral slip

Extensor tendon divided

Distal phalanx

Base of distal phalanx

Head of middle phalanx

a

b

c

Fig. 9.2 Dorsal approach to the proximal distal phalanx, distal interphalangeal joint, and distal middle phalanx. **(a)** Skin incisions; the Y-shaped incision is preferable. **(b)** The skin flaps are retracted with retaining sutures. The exposed extensor tendon is divided distally with a longitudinal, lazy S-shaped incision. **(c)** Exposure of the distal interphalangeal joint.

9.4 Palmar Approach to the Middle Phalanx, Proximal Interphalangeal Joint, and Proximal Phalanx

- Make a zigzag (Bruner) incision on the palmar surface of the finger; reflect the rounded tips of the skin flaps ulnarly or radially at the level of the joint creases (► Fig. 9.3a).

- Expose the flexor tendon sheaths; protect the radial and ulnar neurovascular bundles, which are covered by the Grayson ligaments (► Fig. 9.3b).
- Depending on the approach, incise the tendon sheath laterally close to the insertion, dividing the annular pulleys longitudinally (► Fig. 9.3c).

Practical Tip

Preserve enough tissue for subsequent repair of the annular pulleys.

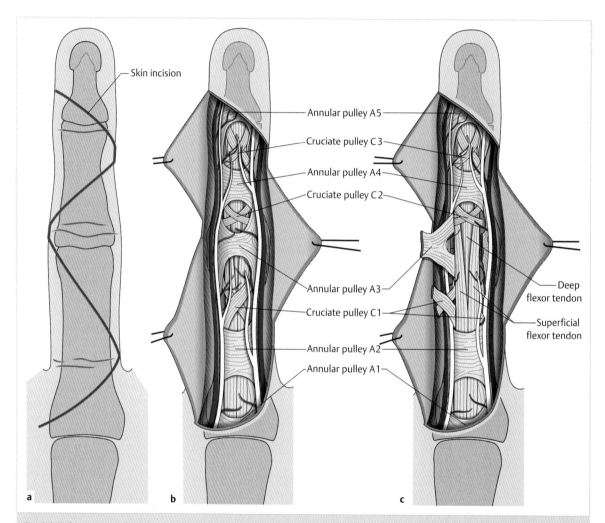

Fig. 9.3 Palmar approach to the middle phalanx, the proximal interphalangeal joint, and the proximal phalanx. **(a)** Zigzag skin incision (Bruner) for surgical exposure of the flexor side of the middle finger. **(b)** Exposure of the tendon sheath, preserving the radial and ulnar neurovascular bundles. A1 to A5: annular pulleys; C1 to C3: cruciate pulleys. **(c)** Palmar exposure of the proximal interphalangeal joint: lateral division of the A3 annular pulley and C1 cruciate pulley, retaining sutures, and exposure of the insertion of the superficial flexor tendon. The A2 annular pulley should be preserved if possible, while the C2 cruciate pulley can be divided if necessary.

- Expose the palmar side of the finger by retracting the flexor tendon.
- To look into the joint, the palmar plate can be divided laterally; subsequent repair must be possible (► Fig. 9.3d).

- Complete exposure of the finger joints is possible only when the lateral ligaments have been detached, preferably distally (► Fig. 9.3e).
- Following hyperextension, the head of the proximal part of the joint can be dislocated fully (► Fig. 9.3f).

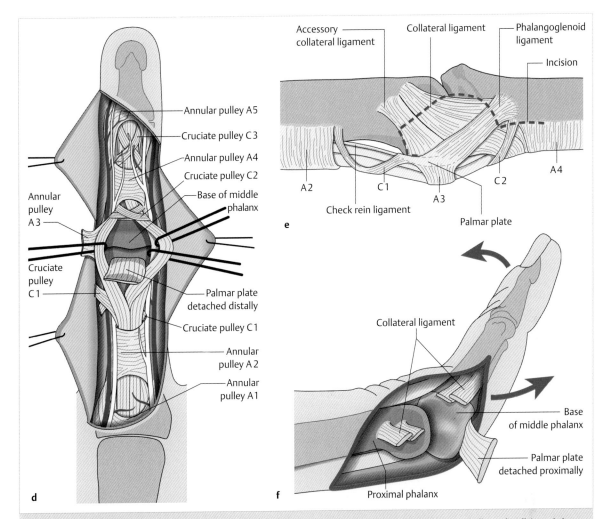

Fig. 9.3 *(Continued)* **(d)** The deep flexor tendon is retracted laterally, the palmar plate is detached (proximally or distally), and the proximal interphalangeal joint is exposed. **(e)** For full exposure of the proximal interphalangeal joint, the collateral ligament is detached on one side (preferably the ulnar side). **(f)** A proximal interphalangeal joint opened by maximum hyperextension and joint dislocation (simplified illustration).

9.5 Dorsal Approach to the Middle and Proximal Phalanx, Proximal Interphalangeal Joint, and Metacarpophalangeal Joint

- Make an S-shaped skin incision, curving around the joints (► Fig. 9.4a),

Practical Tip

Avoid the radial side of the index finger and ulnar side of the little finger.

- Expose the dorsal extensor apparatus, the dorsal aponeurosis, protecting the dorsal sensory nerves (► Fig. 9.4b).
- Access to the middle phalanx shaft (► Fig. 9.4c) is obtained by longitudinal splitting along the center of the distal extensor tendon and triangular lamina (1); an alternative is to divide the transverse retinacular ligament of Landsmeer to expose the middle phalanx by dorsal retraction of the lateral slip (2).
- The approach to the shaft of the proximal phalanx (► Fig. 9.4c) is obtained by longitudinal splitting along the central slip of the extensor tendon (3); an alternative is to make an incision parallel to the central slip or

through the oblique fibers between the central and lateral slips (4); another possibility is to divide the transverse retinacular ligament of Landsmeer, if necessary. The lateral slip of the extensor tendon is retracted dorsally; the oblique fibers of the proximal extensor tendon must then be partially divided longitudinally (5).
- An extended dorsal approach to the proximal interphalangeal joint according to Chamay is obtained by elevation of the central slip of the extensor tendon as a distally based, V-shaped flap (► Fig. 9.4d).

Practical Tip

Avoid a detachment of the extensor central slip on the dorsal base of the middle phalanx.

- The approach to the metacarpophalangeal joint is as follows:
  - By midline splitting of the extensor tendon or parallel to the central slip, preferably dorsoulnar (► Fig. 9.4e).
  - In extended position—possible only from the radial side of the index finger and ulnar side of the little finger—between the collateral ligament and accessory collateral ligament (► Fig. 9.4f).
  - In flexed position—by incision of the dorsal capsule parallel to the collateral ligament (► Fig. 9.4g).

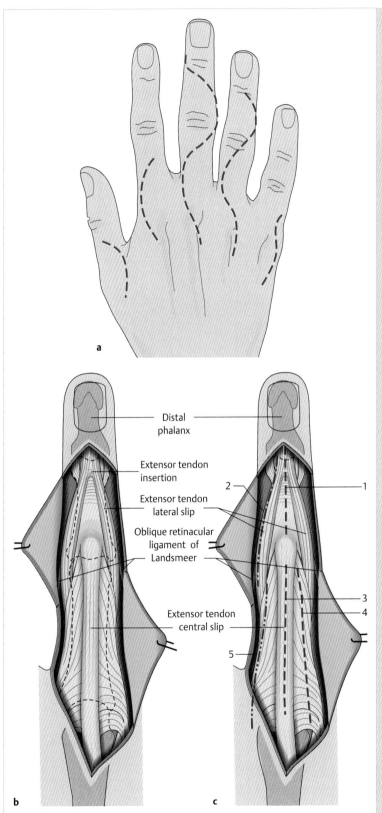

Fig. 9.4 Dorsal approach to the middle and proximal phalanx and to the proximal interphalangeal and metacarpophalangeal joints. **(a)** Skin incisions. **(b)** Exposure of the extensor tendon and dorsal aponeurosis. **(c)** Approach to the shaft of the middle phalanx. 1: central incision through the extensor tendon and triangular lamina; 2: parallel incision along the border of the lateral slip with longitudinal division of the transverse retinacular ligament of Landsmeer. Approach to the shaft of the proximal phalanx. 3: The central slip is split down the middle. 4: A laterally displaced incision is made parallel to the central slip or through the oblique fibers between the central slip and lateral slip. 5: The lateral slip is moved dorsally and, if necessary, the transverse retinacular ligament of Landsmeer and oblique fibers of the proximal extensor apparatus are divided.

Distal phalanx

Extensor tendon insertion

Extensor tendon lateral slip

Oblique retinacular ligament of Landsmeer

Extensor tendon central slip

Continued ▶

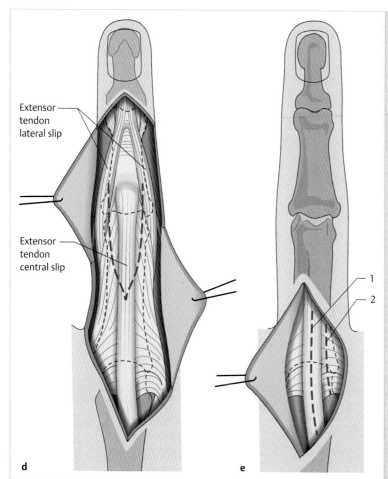

Extensor
tendon
lateral slip

Extensor
tendon
central slip

d

e

1
2

Fig. 9.4 *(Continued)* **(d)** Extended approach to the proximal interphalangeal joint (Chamay). A distally based, V-shaped tendon flap is created by an incision of the central slip. **(e)** Approach to the proximal interphalangeal joint. 1: Longitudinal splitting of the extensor digitorum tendon. 2: Parallel to the central slip, a dorsoulnar incision is made through the oblique fibers between the central and the lateral slips of the extensor tendon.

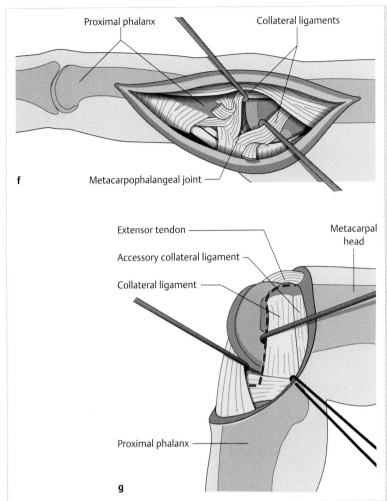

f — Proximal phalanx — Collateral ligaments — Metacarpophalangeal joint

g — Extensor tendon — Accessory collateral ligament — Collateral ligament — Metacarpal head — Proximal phalanx

Fig. 9.4 *(Continued)* **(f)** Approach in extension, between the collateral and accessory collateral ligaments. **(g)** Approach in flexion, by incision of the dorsal capsule parallel to the collateral ligament.

9.6 Mediolateral Approach to the Shaft of Middle Phalanx and Proximal Phalanx, and to Proximal Interphalangeal Joint

- With the finger in maximum flexion, the skin incision is marked on the dorsal flexion crease of each joint (► Fig. 9.5a).
- The finger is then extended and the skin incision joins the marked sites (► Fig. 9.5b); distal and proximal extension at the level of the line is possible.

Practical Tip

The approach should be ulnar on the index finger and radial on the little finger; protect the palmar functional structures, nerves, and vessels.

- Direct approach to the middle phalanx, palmar to the lateral slip, and to the proximal phalanx between the transverse retinacular ligament of Landsmeer and lateral slip (► Fig. 9.5c).
- For better exposure of the proximal phalanx and proximal middle phalanx, the transverse retinacular ligament of Landsmeer is divided, protecting the collateral ligaments of the proximal interphalangeal joint underneath (► Fig. 9.5d).
- Access to the proximal interphalangeal joint after division of the transverse retinacular ligament of Landsmeer is
  ○ dorsal to the collateral ligament (1 in ► Fig. 9.5e);
  ○ in maximum flexion between the collateral ligament and accessory collateral ligament (2 in ► Fig. 9.5e); and/or
  ○ between the accessory ligament and palmar plate (3 in ► Fig. 9.5e).

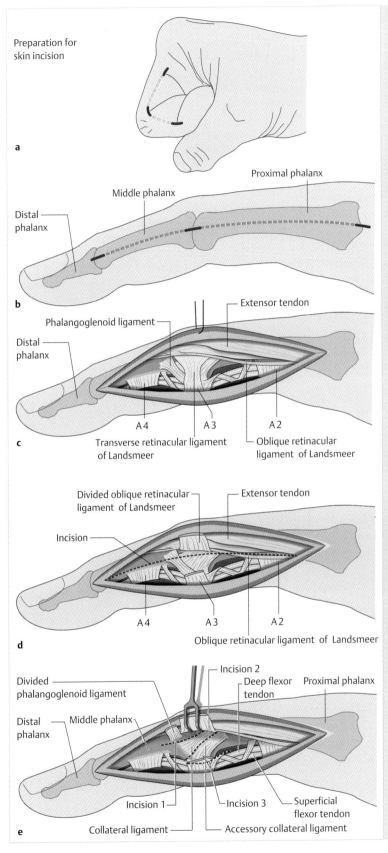

Preparation for skin incision

a

Proximal phalanx

Middle phalanx

Distal phalanx

b

Phalangoglenoid ligament

Extensor tendon

Distal phalanx

A 4

A 3

A 2

Transverse retinacular ligament of Landsmeer

Oblique retinacular ligament of Landsmeer

c

Divided oblique retinacular ligament of Landsmeer

Extensor tendon

Incision

A 4

A 3

A 2

Oblique retinacular ligament of Landsmeer

d

Divided phalangoglenoid ligament

Incision 2

Deep flexor tendon

Proximal phalanx

Distal phalanx

Middle phalanx

Incision 1

Incision 3

Superficial flexor tendon

Collateral ligament

Accessory collateral ligament

e

Fig. 9.5 Mediolateral approach to the shaft of the middle and proximal phalanx and to the proximal interphalangeal and metacarpophalangeal joints. (a) Preparation of the skin incision for the mediolateral approach to the middle and proximal phalanges and their joints. Maximum flexion of the finger produces joint grooves, the dorsal ends of which are marked as shown. (b) The finger is extended and the skin markings are joined by a straight line. The skin incision is made along this line. (c) The lateral extensor apparatus: the central and lateral slips are exposed. (d) Division of the transverse retinacular ligament of Landsmeer allows direct access to the middle and proximal phalanx. (e) The approach to the proximal interphalangeal joint is either dorsal to the collateral ligament (1), in maximum flexion between the collateral ligament and accessory collateral ligament (2), or most clearly between the accessory collateral ligament and the palmar plate (3).

9.7 Dorsal Approach to the Metacarpals

- A straight or S-shaped skin incision is made on the extensor surface of the hand; a straight incision should run parallel to but not directly over the extensor tendons (▶ Fig. 9.6a).

> **Caution**
>
> Protect dorsal sensory nerves and longitudinally running veins.

- Retract the extensor tendons laterally; expose the interosseous muscles and detach them partially; if possible, preserve the intertendinous connections (▶ Fig. 9.6b).
- The approach to the base of the fifth metacarpal is through a dorsoulnar incision moved radially (▶ Fig. 9.6c).
- The dorsal sensory branch of the ulnar nerve must be exposed and protected; the tendons of the little finger are retracted laterally (▶ Fig. 9.6d).
- The muscles of the little finger sometimes have to be partially detached.

9.8 Approaches to the Thumb

- The palmar (▶ Fig. 9.7a top right), dorsal (▶ Fig. 9.7a top bottom), and mediolateral (▶ Fig. 9.7a top left) approaches for distal and proximal phalanx, the interphalangeal joint, the metacarpophalangeal joint, and the metacarpal shaft correspond to those for the fingers.
- The dorsoulnar approach to the metacarpophalangeal joint is moved ulnarward by means of an incision parallel to the extensor tendon (▶ Fig. 9.7a top left); alternatively, an ulnar curved, palmar convex incision (▶ Fig. 9.7a lower dot-dashline), or a, dorsally convex (▶ Fig. 9.7a lower dashedline) may be made.
- With the dorsoulnar approach, the tendons of extensor pollicis brevis and longus and the aponeurosis of adductor pollicis are exposed, protecting the dorsoulnar sensory branch of the nerve (▶ Fig. 9.7b).
- The extensor tendons and adductor pollicis aponeurosis are exposed and the adductor insertion is incised parallel to the extensor tendons (▶ Fig. 9.7c).
- The metacarpophalangeal joint is opened by dorsoulnar incision of the joint capsule (▶ Fig. 9.7d).

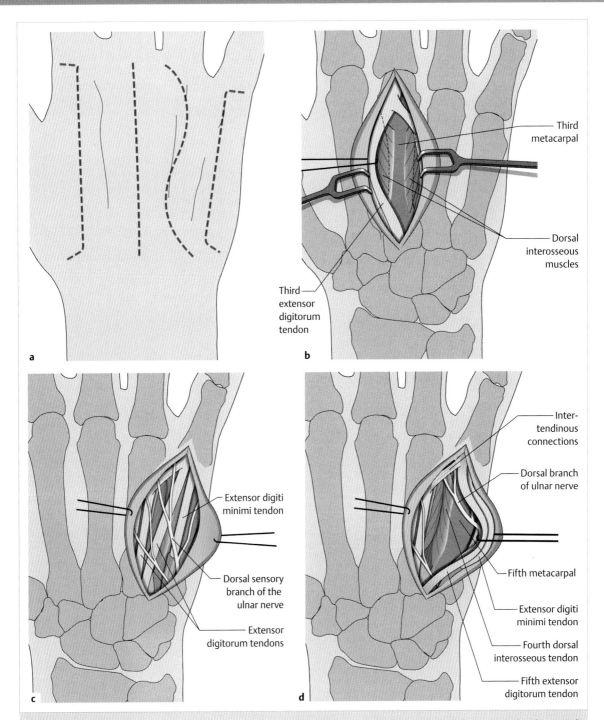

Fig. 9.6 Dorsal approach to the metacarpals. **(a)** Straight or S-shaped skin incisions. **(b)** The extensor tendon is exposed and retracted, giving direct dorsal access to the metacarpal. Partial detachment of the interosseous muscles from the bone. **(c)** Approach to the dorsum of the fifth metacarpal: straight incision on the radial side with careful exposure of the dorsal sensory branch of the ulnar nerve. **(d)** The extensor tendon and nerve branch are retracted ulnarward, giving direct access to the fifth metacarpal.

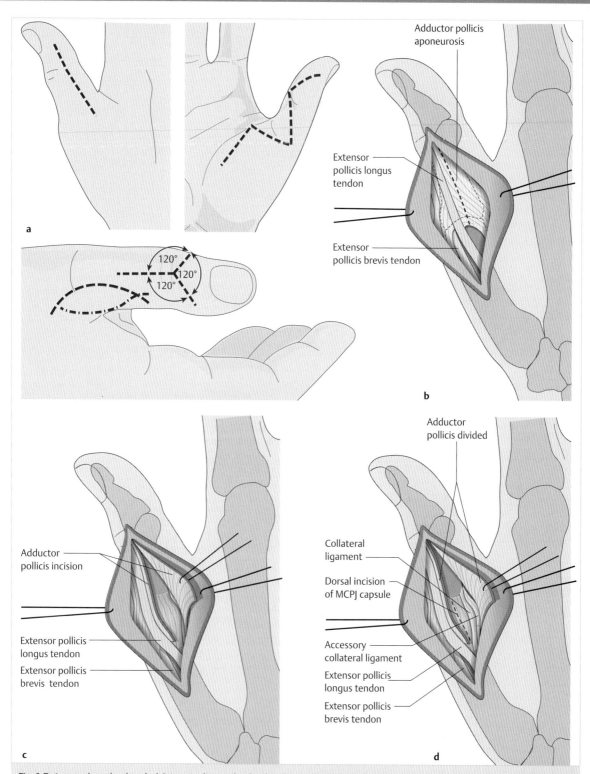

Fig. 9.7 Approach to the thumb. **(a)** Approaches to the distal and proximal phalanx and the metacarpal of the thumb. The mediolateral, palmar, and dorsal skin incisions correspond to those of the fingers. **(b)** In the dorsoulnar approach to the metacarpophalangeal joint, after skin incision (see Fig. 9.7a), the extensor pollicis longus and brevis tendons and the aponeurosis of adductor pollicis are exposed. **(c)** Incision of the adductor pollicis insertion is performed parallel to the extensor tendon, which is then retracted. **(d)** Exposure of the ulnar collateral ligament and opening of the joint for inspection through a dorsal incision of the capsule. MCPJ, metacarpophalangeal joint.

9.9 Approach to the Carpo (trapezio-)metacarpal Joint (According to Moberg, Gedda and Wagner)

- The skin incision passes proximally from the distal dorsoulnar third of the first metacarpal and curves in a semicircle to the palmar side of the thenar eminence at the level of the trapezium; alternatively, it may be S-shaped, passing in proximal palmar direction around the scaphoid tubercle to the tendon of flexor carpi radialis (► Fig. 9.8a, b).

Caution

Preserve the superficial branches of the radial nerve and the dorsal branch of the radial artery.

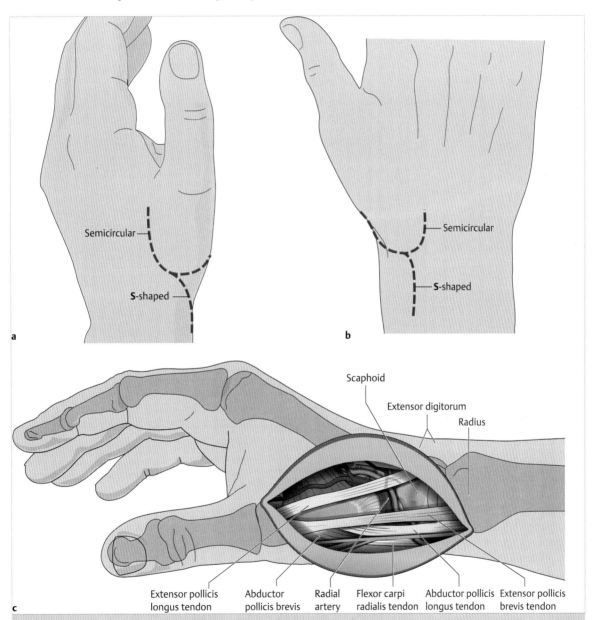

Fig. 9.8 Approach to the first carpo(trapezio)metacarpal joint. **(a)** Dorsal skin incisions. **(b)** Radial skin incisions. **(c)** Exposure of the abductor pollicis longus and extensor pollicis brevis tendons, flexor carpi radialis tendon sheath, and the dorsal branch of the radial artery.

Continued ▶

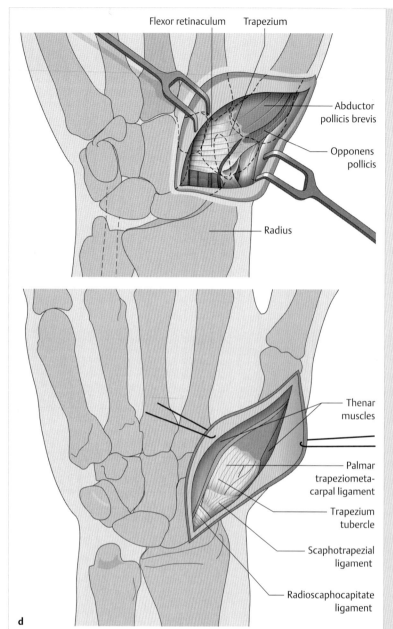

Flexor retinaculum   Trapezium

Abductor pollicis brevis

Opponens pollicis

Radius

Thenar muscles

Palmar trapeziometa-carpal ligament

Trapezium tubercle

Scaphotrapezial ligament

Radioscaphocapitate ligament

d

Fig. 9.8 *(Continued)* **(d)** After partial detachment of the muscles from the base of the first metacarpal and the palmar side of the trapezium, the palmar ligaments of the carpo(trapezio)metacarpal joint are exposed. Access to the joint is through a transverse or **T**-shaped division of the ligaments.

- The insertion of abductor pollicis brevis and flexor pollicis brevis is partly divided from the base of the first metacarpal and the palmar surface of the trapezium (▶ Fig. 9.8c).

- Exposed ligaments at the base of the first metacarpal and trapezium are divided transversely or longitudinally to open the carpometacarpal joint (▶ Fig. 9.8d).

9.10 Palmar Approach to the Wrist

- An **S**-shaped incision is made parallel to the thenar crease of the thenar eminence, which can be extended distally and proximally (▶ Fig. 9.9a), preserving the palmar branch of the median nerve.
- The flexor retinaculum is exposed and the carpal tunnel is opened ulnar to the palmaris longus tendon and radial to the hook of the hamate (▶ Fig. 9.9b); the course of the median nerve may show variations as well as the thenar branch of the median nerve.
- The superficial palmar arterial arch is exposed; all of the flexor tendons and the median nerve are mobilized and retracted laterally as necessary.
- The palmar wrist ligaments are exposed (▶ Fig. 9.9c).

Note

The palmar radioulnar ligament should be preserved whenever possible to avoid instability of the distal radioulnar joint.

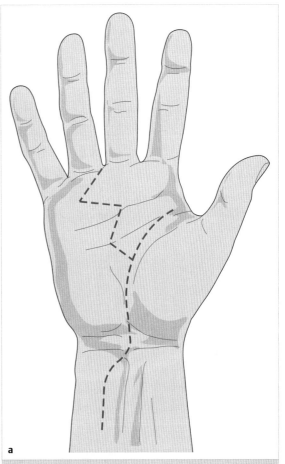

a

Fig. 9.9 Palmar approach to the wrist. **(a)** An S-shaped skin incision parallel to the thenar eminence with zigzag proximal and distal extensions as needed.

Continued ▶

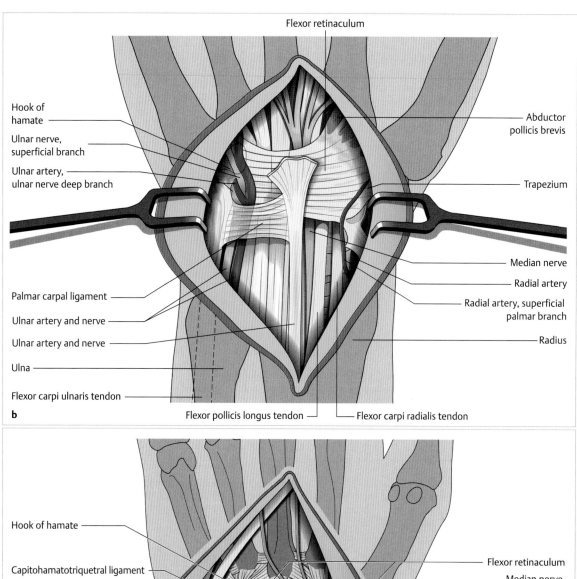

Flexor retinaculum

Hook of hamate

Ulnar nerve, superficial branch

Ulnar artery, ulnar nerve deep branch

Abductor pollicis brevis

Trapezium

Median nerve

Radial artery

Radial artery, superficial palmar branch

Radius

Palmar carpal ligament

Ulnar artery and nerve

Ulnar artery and nerve

Ulna

Flexor carpi ulnaris tendon

b

Flexor pollicis longus tendon

Flexor carpi radialis tendon

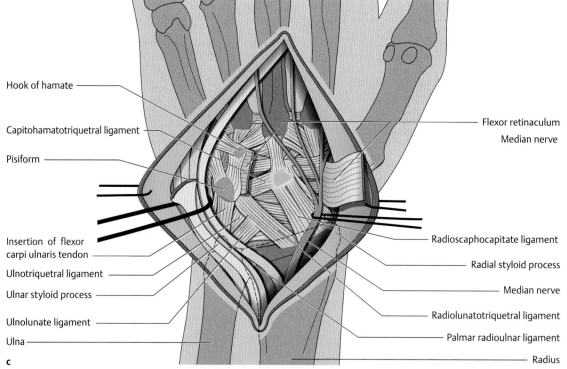

Hook of hamate

Capitohamatotriquetral ligament

Pisiform

Flexor retinaculum

Median nerve

Insertion of flexor carpi ulnaris tendon

Ulnotriquetral ligament

Ulnar styloid process

Ulnolunate ligament

Ulna

c

Radioscaphocapitate ligament

Radial styloid process

Median nerve

Radiolunatotriquetral ligament

Palmar radioulnar ligament

Radius

Fig. 9.9 *(Continued)* **(b)** Exposure of the palmaris longus tendon and flexor retinaculum. The carpal tunnel is opened by longitudinal incision of the retinaculum ulnar to the palmaris longus tendon and just radial to the hook of the hamate. The median nerve is exposed and the thenar branch is identified. The flexor tendons are exposed and retracted laterally, and the superficial palmar arch is dissected. **(c)** Exposure of the palmar carpal ligaments.

9.11 Dorsal Approach to the Wrist

- The straight skin incision passes proximally from the base of the third metacarpal ulnar to Lister's tubercle. Alternatively, a straight incision from the base of the second metacarpal passes proximally and ulnarward to the distal end of the ulna at a distance of approximately the width of two fingers (▶ Fig. 9.10a).

- Expose the extensor retinaculum from the second to fifth extensor compartment; on the radial side, look out for the superficial branch of the radial nerve (▶ Fig. 9.10b).

- Open the second and third extensor tendon compartments to expose the extensor tendons; open the fourth and fifth extensor compartments from the radial side, then retract the extensor tendons (▶ Fig. 9.10c).
- Expose the dorsal carpal ligament system. Depending on the type of injury, make either a longitudinal / T-shaped incision (▶ Fig. 9.10d), or a distally pedicled U-shaped incision (▶ Fig. 9.10e), or radially pedicled U-shaped incision (▶ Fig. 9.10f) in the ligament apparatus.

Practical Tip

Do not split the dorsal radioulnar ligament. A sufficiently large piece of the radiolunotriquetral ligament must be left on the radius to allow for subsequent repair. Transosseous repair may be performed as an alternative.

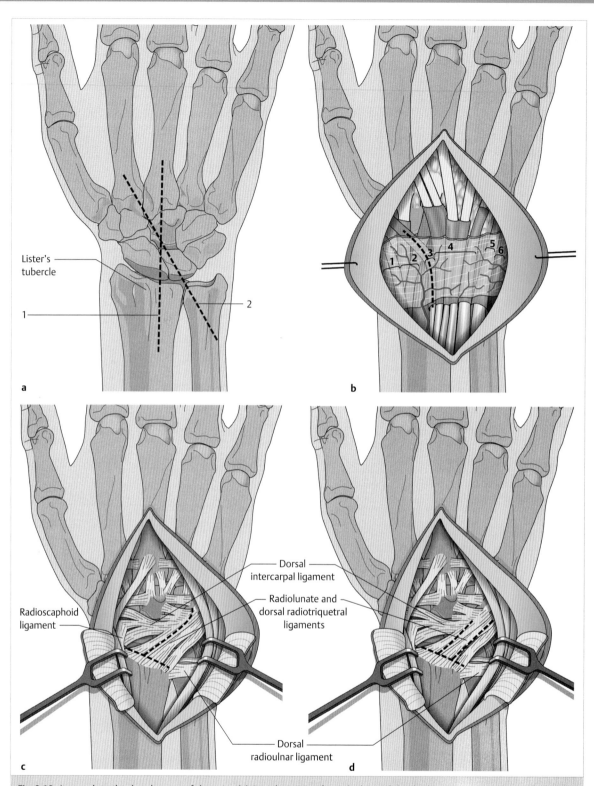

Lister's tubercle

1

2

a

b

Radioscaphoid ligament

Dorsal intercarpal ligament

Radiolunate and dorsal radiotriquetral ligaments

Dorsal radioulnar ligament

c

d

Fig. 9.10 Approach to the dorsal aspect of the wrist. **(a)** Straight incision from the base of the third metacarpal to Lister's tubercle (1). Variant: straight incision from the base of the second metacarpal ulnarward, proximal to the styloid process of the ulna (2). **(b)** Exposure of the extensor retinaculum with the first to fifth extensor tendon compartments. **(c)** The second, third, and also the fourth and fifth extensor compartments are opened, creating radially and ulnarly based retinaculum flaps. The extensor tendons are retracted laterally; if possible do not touch the 6th extensor tendon compartment. **(d)** The dorsal ligament apparatus is exposed, identified and incised longitudinally or in T-shape to form flaps.

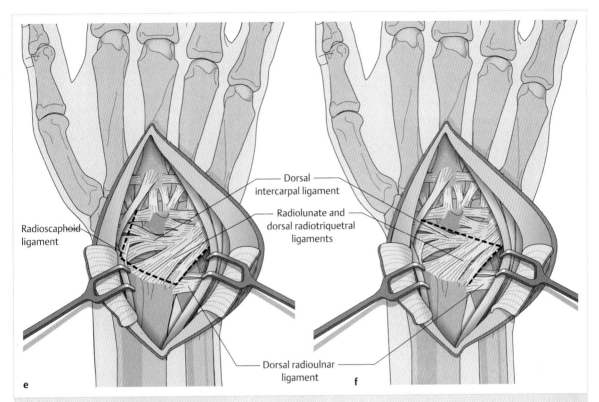

Radioscaphoid ligament

Dorsal intercarpal ligament

Radiolunate and dorsal radiotriquetral ligaments

Dorsal radioulnar ligament

e

f

Fig. 9.10 (*Continued*) (**e**) Incision and creation of distally based U-shaped flap. (**f**) Incision and creation of radially based U-shaped flap.

9.12 Radiopalmar Approach to the Wrist and Scaphoid

- A hockey stick incision is made from the scaphoid tubercle to the palpable tendon sheath of flexor carpi radialis with proximal extension next to the tendon sheath (▶ Fig. 9.11a). The superficial branch of the radial artery may be ligated if necessary.
- After longitudinal incision of the tendon sheath, the tendon of flexor carpi radialis is retracted ulnarward (▶ Fig. 9.11b).

⚠ Caution

Palmar branch of the median nerve.

- Longitudinal incision from distal to proximal of the radioscaphocapitate ligament (▶ Fig. 9.11c).

Practical Tip

To preserve the blood supply to the proximal pole of the scaphoid, keep the proximal extension-incision as short as possible.

- The distal pole of the scaphoid is exposed by longitudinal division of the thenar muscles.
- If the approach is extended to expose the distal pole of the scaphoid, make a T-shaped incision in the radiolunotriquetral ligament (▶ Fig. 9.11c, d).

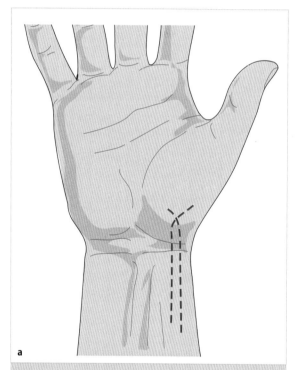

Fig. 9.11 Radiopalmar approach to the scaphoid.
(a) Straight or slightly hockey stick incision proximally, from the scaphoid tubercle toward the flexor carpi radialis tendon sheath. Caution: palmar branch of median nerve.

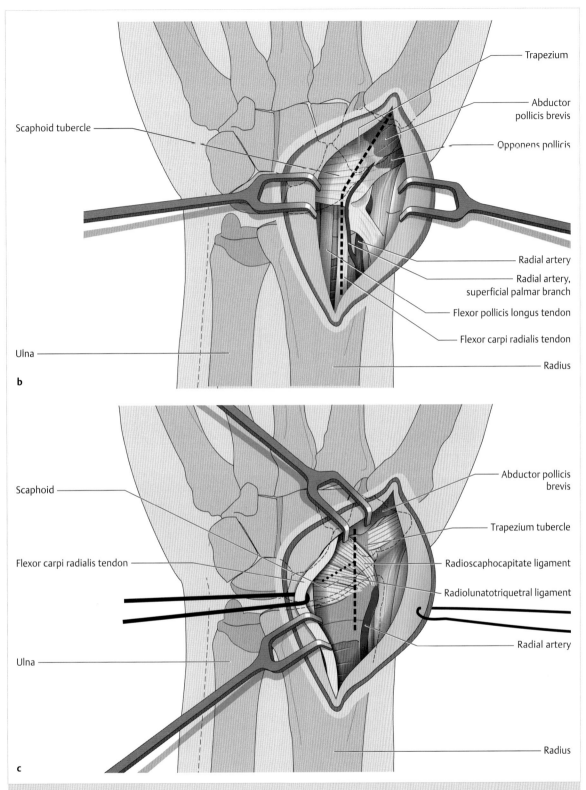

Trapezium

Abductor pollicis brevis

Opponens pollicis

Scaphoid tubercle

Radial artery

Radial artery, superficial palmar branch

Flexor pollicis longus tendon

Flexor carpi radialis tendon

Ulna

Radius

b

Abductor pollicis brevis

Scaphoid

Trapezium tubercle

Flexor carpi radialis tendon

Radioscaphocapitate ligament

Radiolunatotriquetral ligament

Ulna

Radial artery

Radius

c

Fig. 9.11 (*Continued*) **(b)** Longitudinal incision of the flexor carpi radialis tendon sheath and ulnarward retraction of the tendon. **(c)** Longitudinal incision of the radioscaphocapitate ligament and partial detachment of the short thenar muscles. If necessary, access to the carpal bones can be extended by a T-shaped incision of the radiolunotriquetral ligament.

Continued ▶

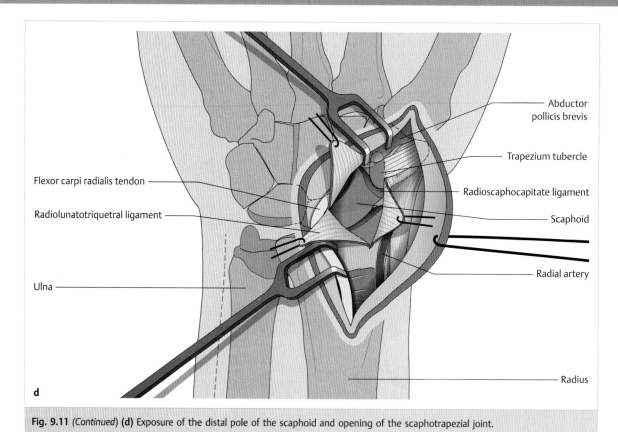

Fig. 9.11 *(Continued)* **(d)** Exposure of the distal pole of the scaphoid and opening of the scaphotrapezial joint.

9.13 Radiodorsal Approach to the Wrist / Proximal Scaphoid Pole

- The longitudinal skin incision passes distally from Lister's tubercle to the base of the third metacarpal, preserving the superficial branch of the radial nerve (▶ Fig. 9.12a); or, alternatively, a transverse lazy S-shaped (black dashed line) or transverse straight incision (red dashed line) may be made.
- The extensor retinaculum is exposed and the third extensor tendon compartment is opened over the tendon of extensor pollicis longus (▶ Fig. 9.12b).

- The tendon is retracted radially with the tendons of the second extensor compartment; the dorsal ligament apparatus is exposed and incised in the direction of the fibers of the dorsal radiolunate ligament, starting from the dorsal border of the radius. If necessary, the approach is extended by an additional incision in radial direction (▶ Fig. 9.12c, d).
- With the wrist in maximum flexion, the scaphoid pole is exposed proximally, along with the scapholunate ligament and the radial side of the lunate (▶ Fig. 9.12e).

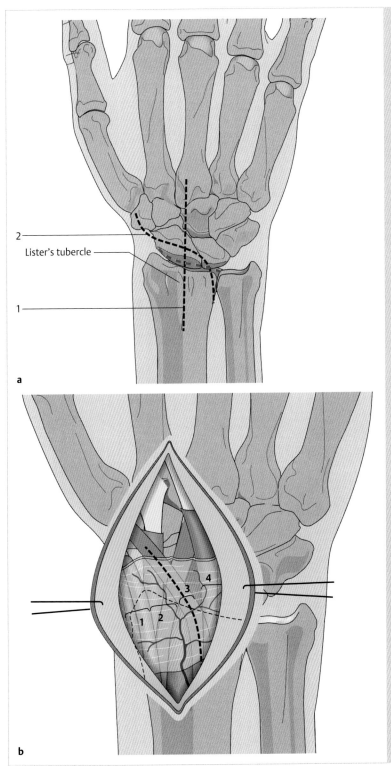

2

Lister's tubercle

1

a

b

Fig. 9.12 Radiodorsal approach to the scaphoid. **(a)** Skin incision from Lister's tubercle distally toward the base of the third metacarpal. **(b)** Exposure and opening of the third extensor tendon compartment and exposure of the tendon of extensor pollicis longus.

Continued ▶

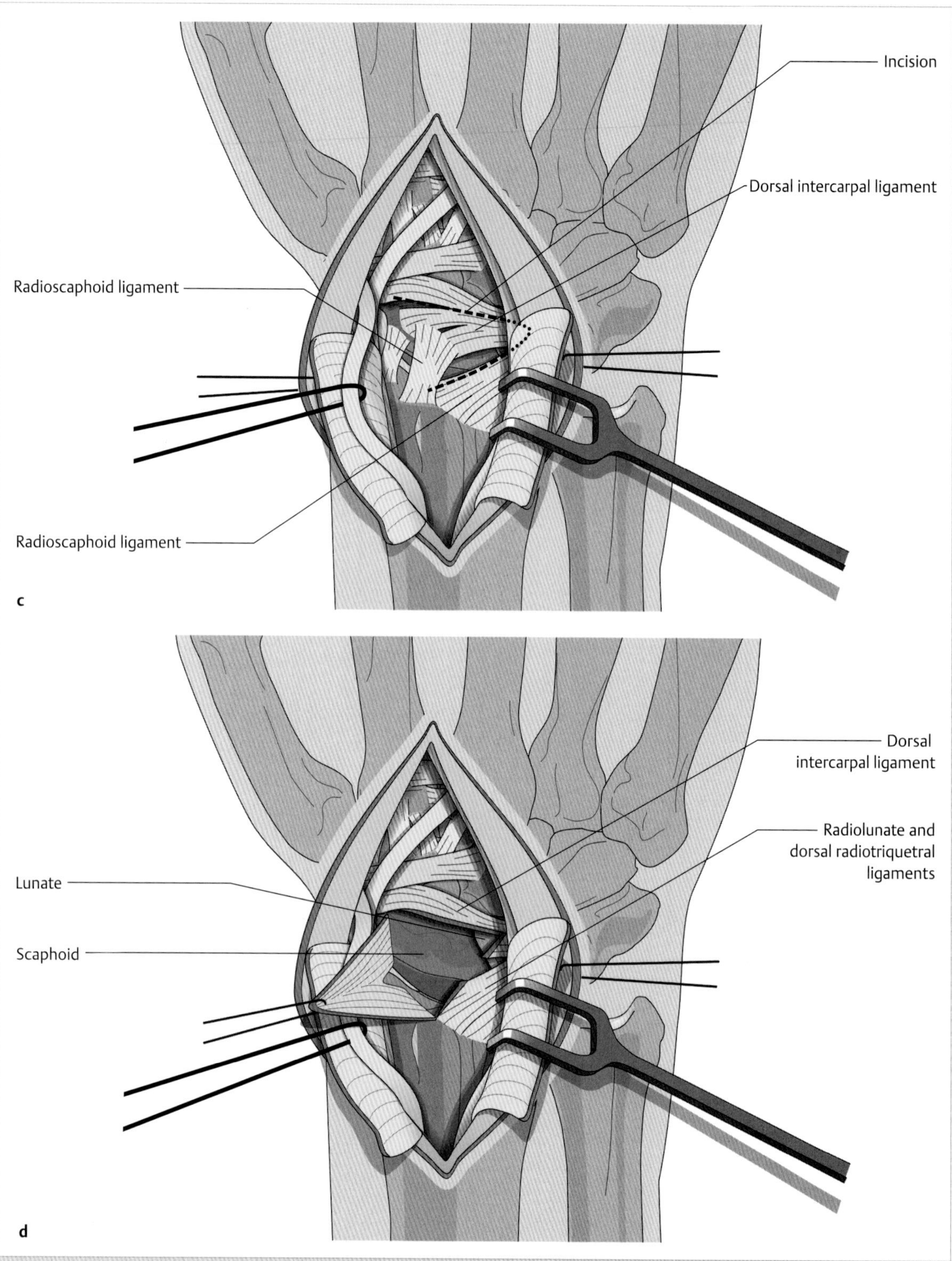

Incision

Dorsal intercarpal ligament

Radioscaphoid ligament

Radioscaphoid ligament

c

Dorsal intercarpal ligament

Radiolunate and dorsal radiotriquetral ligaments

Lunate

Scaphoid

d

Fig. 9.12 (*Continued*) (**c**) Exposure of the radioscaphoid and radiolunate ligaments. The capsule is incised parallel to the direction of the fibers. (**d**) The radially based ligament and capsule flap are reflected radially.

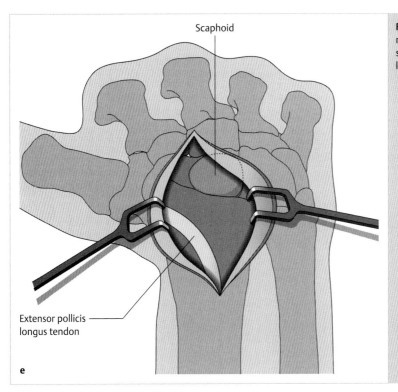

Scaphoid

Extensor pollicis
longus tendon

e

Fig. 9.12 (Continued) (e) With the wrist in
maximum flexion, the proximal pole of the
scaphoid is exposed and the scapholunate
ligament comes into view.

9.14 Dorsal Ulnar Approach to the Wrist (Triquetrum, Hamate, Ulnar Midcarpal Joints)

- The skin incision passes from the base of the fifth metacarpal proximally around the radial side of the distal ulna, extending it proximally parallel to the ulnar shaft, exposing carefully the dorsal sensory branch of the ulnar nerve (▶ Fig. 9.13a).
- The extensor retinaculum is exposed and the fifth extensor tendon compartment is split longitudinally. If necessary, the fourth extensor compartment is opened on the ulnar side; the extensor tendons of the little finger are retracted ulnarly, and the tendons of the fourth compartment are retracted radially (▶ Fig. 9.13b).

Practical Tip

If possible, avoid the sixth extensor compartment. If necessary, detach the sixth compartment from the ulna, together with the periosteum, so that the tendon of extensor carpi ulnaris remains in the tendon sheath.

- The dorsal wrist ligaments are incised parallel to the dorsal radiotriquetral ligament, with ulnodorsal proximal extension parallel to the tendon of extensor carpi ulnaris (▶ Fig. 9.13c).
- If necessary for exposure of the lunatotriquetral joint, a T-shaped incision is made in the dorsal radiotriquetral ligament, preserving the dorsal radioulnar ligament (▶ Fig. 9.13c).
- To expose the TFCC (triangular fibrocartilage complex) make a transverse incision in the ulnar carpal joint parallel and distal to the dorsal radioulnar ligament.
- To expose the ulnar midcarpal bones, incise the dorsal intercarpal ligament in the direction of its fibers distal to the triquetrum, then make an incision parallel to the fibers along the ulnar border of the dorsal radiotriquetral ligament to create a radially based, V-shaped ligamentous flap (▶ Fig. 9.13c, d).

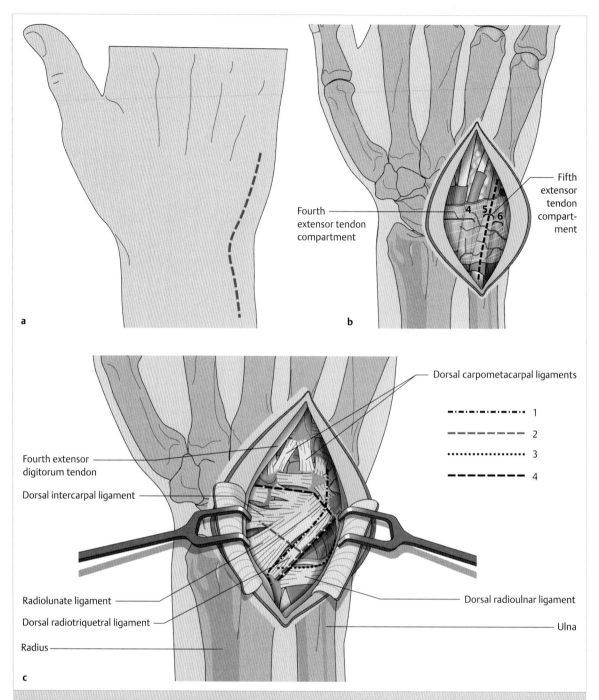

Fifth
extensor
tendon
compart-
ment

Fourth
extensor tendon
compartment

4 5 6

a

b

Dorsal carpometacarpal ligaments

1

2

3

4

Fourth extensor
digitorum tendon

Dorsal intercarpal ligament

Radiolunate ligament

Dorsal radiotriquetral ligament

Radius

Dorsal radioulnar ligament

Ulna

c

Fig. 9.13 Dorsal ulnar approach to the wrist. **(a)** Skin incision from the base of the fifth metacarpal passing proximally around the styloid process of the ulna. **(b)** Exposure of the fourth and fifth compartments of the extensor retinaculum. **(c)** Exposure of the dorsal carpal ligament system. Incision parallel to the fibers of the dorsal radiotriquetral ligament (1), and proximal extension parallel to the tendon of flexor carpi ulnaris. To expose the lunotriquetral joint, a T-shaped incision must be made in the dorsal radiotriquetral ligament (2). To expose the TFCC (triangular fibrocartilage complex), a transverse incision is made in the dorsal joint capsule parallel and distal to the radioulnar ligament (3). To expose the ulnar midcarpal joint, capitate, hamate, and triquetrum, an additional incision is made parallel to the direction of the fibers of the dorsal intercarpal ligament and this creates a radially based ligamentous flap (4).

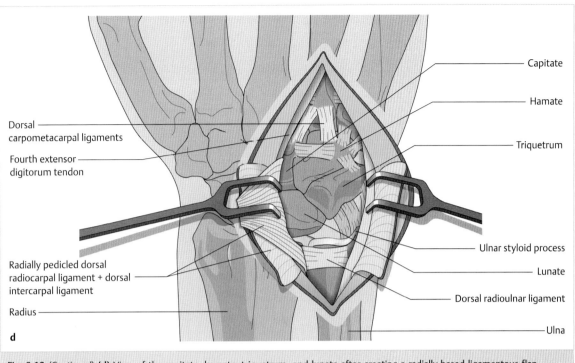

Capitate

Hamate

Triquetrum

Dorsal carpometacarpal ligaments

Fourth extensor digitorum tendon

Ulnar styloid process

Lunate

Radially pedicled dorsal radiocarpal ligament + dorsal intercarpal ligament

Dorsal radioulnar ligament

Radius

Ulna

d

Fig. 9.13 (*Continued*) **(d)** View of the capitate, hamate, triquetrum, and lunate after creating a radially based ligamentous flap.

Chapter 10

Surgical Procedures

10

10 Surgical Procedures

10.1 Overview

Uncomplicated fracture healing after open reduction and internal fixation requires stable fixation. Only then does the advantage of operative therapy become apparent, namely, early *active motion stability*.

Secondary fracture healing is achieved with closed reduction and fixation using percutaneous operation methods, which usually require additional temporary postoperative external immobilization or an external fixator.

The following are commonly employed operation methods:

- Wire suture
- Tension band wiring
- Lag screw(s)
- Lag screw plus neutralization plate
- Percutaneous lag screw
- Plate fixation:
  - Standard plate
  - Dynamic compression plate
  - Hybrid plate
- Fixed-angle locking plate
- Condylar plate
- Intraosseous compression:
  - Intraosseous screw, headless bone screw (HBS)
  - Intraosseous compression wire
- Intramedullary Kirschner wire or pin
- External fixator
- Adaptive fixation:
  - Percutaneous Kirschner wire fixation
  - Hooked wire
  - Plugging method
  - Retrograde wire drilling
  - Ishiguro operation / extension-block pinning
  - Transfixation
- Temporary joint transfixation
- Dynamic distraction external fixation
- Pull-out barbed wire suture / Lengemann
- Hooked plate
- Absorbable pins

10.2 Wire Suture

10.2.1 Procedure

- Drill two holes, approximately 1 cm proximal and 1 cm distal to the fracture gap, transverse to the shaft axis (Fig. 10.1a)
- The drill holes should be dorsal to the long midlateral axis (▶ Fig. 10.1b) with a diameter of 1 mm.
- Thread two wires (diameter 0.8 mm) through the holes.

- Twist the wires together at the level of the fracture (▶ Fig. 10.1d), tightening them equally on both sides.

Practical Tip

Pass a size no. 1 needle through the drill hole and introduce the 0.8-mm wire into the tip of the needle. Advance the wire and withdraw the needle (▶ Fig. 10.1c)

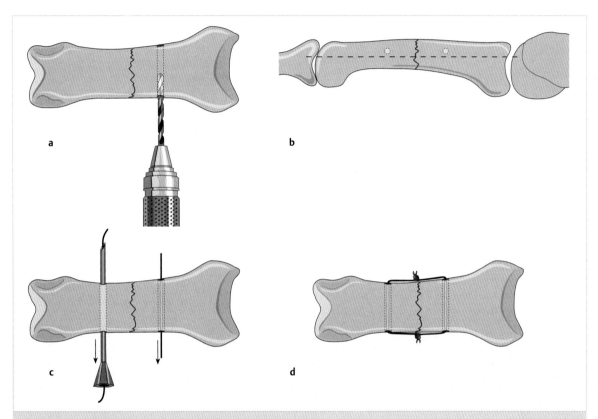

Fig. 10.1 Wire suture. **(a)** Two holes are drilled transversely to the shaft axis, 1 cm proximal and 1 cm distal to the fracture. **(b)** The drill holes are dorsal to the long axis of the bone. **(c)** A sufficiently large needle is pushed into the hole, the wire is pushed through the needle, and the needle is removed. The procedure is repeated in the second hole. **(d)** The two wires are twisted together at the level of the fracture by pulling evenly on both at the same time.

10.3 Tension Band Wiring

▶ **Principle.** When fractures are located in the area of bending forces, tension band wiring can generate inter-fragmental compression on loading. The fixation material must be placed on the side exposed to tensile forces. Compression is then produced on the bending side. By means of this intertragmental compression, the fracture usually heals.

▶ **Application.** Tension band wiring—applied to the extensor side in the middle third—is effective for transverse fractures of the metacarpals. Tension banding is also useful for avulsion and traction fractures. In this case, the fixation neutralizes the pull of the tendons on the avulsed fragment. The method is used most frequently for intra-articular avulsion fractures such as the type III Busch fracture of the proximal end of the distal phalanx and intra-articular fracture of the base of the fifth metacarpal.

10.3.1 Shaft Fractures

- Drill two holes transversely, approximately 1 cm proximal and 1 cm distal to the fracture gap (▶ Fig. 10.2a).
- The drill holes are palmar to the long midlateral axis, diameter 1 mm (▶ Fig. 10.2b).
- Thread two wires (diameter 0.8 mm) through the holes using a size no. 1 needle.
- Draw one of the wires along the extensor side of the bone on the periosteum palmar to the extensor tendon to the contralateral hole located beyond the fracture (▶ Fig. 10.2c).

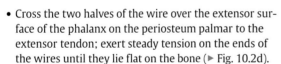

Caution

Handle the extensor tendon gently.

- Cross the two halves of the wire over the extensor surface of the phalanx on the periosteum palmar to the extensor tendon; exert steady tension on the ends of the wires until they lie flat on the bone (▶ Fig. 10.2d).
- The ends of the first wire are twisted together with the ends of the second wire with steady tension distal or proximal to the fracture gap (▶ Fig. 10.2e).

- For additional fracture stabilization, a Kirschner wire may be inserted obliquely, diameter 1 mm (▶ Fig. 10.2f), but only after completing the tension band wiring. This is usually not necessary, however.

10.3.2 Intra-articular Avulsion or Traction Fractures

- Make a Y-shaped skin incision over the dorsum of the distal interphalangeal joint (▶ Fig. 9.2).
- Expose the dorsal intra-articular fracture of the base of the distal phalanx and clean the fracture gap.
- Expose the shaft of the distal phalanx bilaterally, if possible as far laterally as the midlateral line. Drill transversely through the distal phalanx shaft (▶ Fig. 10.3a).
- Exchange the drill for a needle with a sufficiently large lumen.
- Insert a tension band wire through the needle and withdraw the needle. The wire remains in the shaft of the distal phalanx with the ends projecting on both sides (▶ Fig. 10.3b).
- The fracture is reduced and fixed by parallel Kirschner wires in the opposite palmar cortex.
- Wire loops are placed proximally around the two Kirschner wires (▶ Fig. 10.3c); alternatively, a needle can be advanced transversely palmar to the extensor tendon insertion directly at the base of the dorsal rim/avulsion fragment of the distal phalanx (▶ Fig. 10.3d).
- After placing the distal tension band wire ends in a figure of **8**, they are twisted evenly with the proximal tension band wire on either side to compress the fracture (▶ Fig. 10.3e).
- The projecting Kirschner wires are bent and shortened so that they can be buried subcutaneously. The skin is sutured.

Note

The tension band wires must be tightened symmetrically with care so as to avoid fracturing the avulsion fragment.

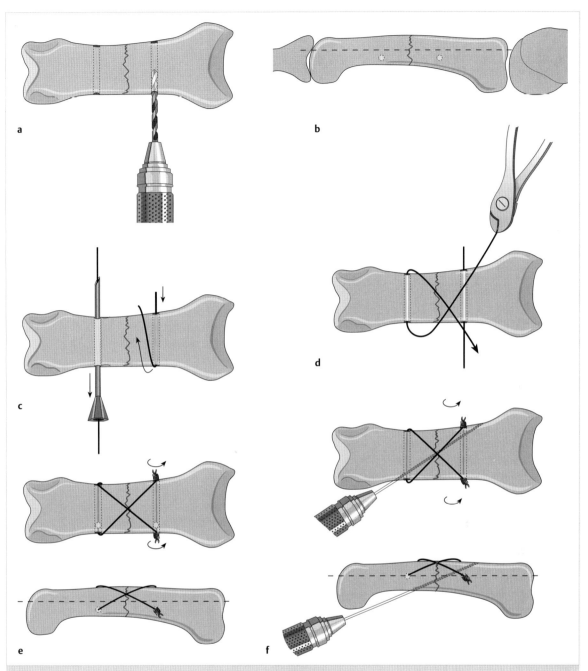

Fig. 10.2 Tension band wiring of a shaft fracture. **(a)** Two holes are drilled transversely to the shaft axis, approximately 1 cm proximal and 1 cm distal to the fracture. **(b)** The drill holes are located palmar to the long axis of the bone. **(c)** Two wires are threaded through the drill holes (see tip in Chapter 10.2.1). **(d)** One tension band wire is pulled through in a cruciate pattern to the contralateral drill hole, dorsal to the fracture but palmar to the extensor tendon and lying directly on the periosteum. **(e)** The ends of the wires are twisted together proximal or distal to the fracture under steady traction. **(f)** If the tension banding is not stable enough, a Kirschner wire can be inserted obliquely to bridge the fracture.

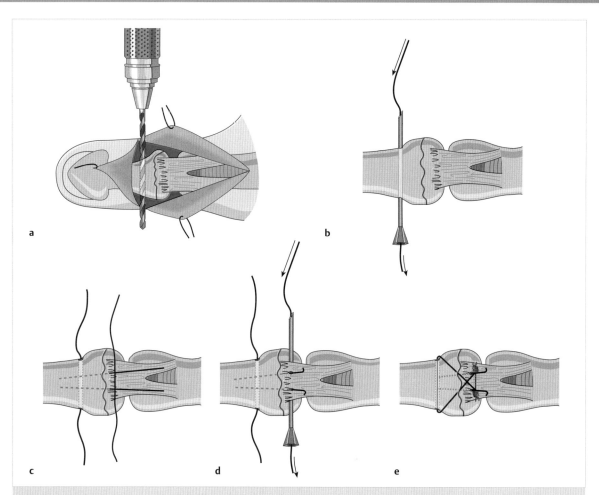

Fig. 10.3 Tension band wiring of an avulsion fracture. **(a)** After a Y-shaped incision over the dorsum of the distal interphalangeal joint, the fracture is exposed and cleaned. The shaft of the distal phalanx is exposed bilaterally as far as the palmar/dorsal midline. The distal phalanx shaft is drilled transversely. **(b)** The drill is exchanged for a needle with an internal diameter greater than the outer diameter of the tension band wire. The wire is pulled through the needle and removed by drawing it over the wire. The wire must project sufficiently on both sides. **(c)** The fracture is reduced and fixed by two parallel Kirschner wires, which are fixed in the opposite cortex. A second tension band wire is placed proximally around the Kirschner wires over the extensor tendon. **(d)** Alternatively, a needle can be pushed transversely close to the dorsal bony edge of the base of the distal phalanx. The needle is passed palmar to the extensor tendon insertion. A second tension band wire is threaded through and the needle is withdrawn, leaving the wire in place. **(e)** The distal tension band wire is placed in a figure-of-8 so that it crosses on the dorsum of the shaft of the distal phalanx. It is twisted with the proximal wire bilaterally, producing interfragmental compression in the fracture. The two Kirschner wires are bent, shortened, and compressed, and the ends are buried subcutaneously by suturing the skin.

10.4 Lag Screw

Internal fixation with a lag screw is an effective method for obtaining functional stable fixation of oblique and torsional fractures. Moreover, lag screws are used for fixation of avulsion fractures and intra-articular metaphyseal fractures. The joint surface is restored without a step-off through interfragmental compression.

In addition a neutralization plate is usually necessary to absorb external forces acting on the fracture in order to achieve, at least, relative stability (see Chapter 10.5.1).

Percutaneous lag screw fixation through stab incisions is possible with special instruments, which helps to minimize soft tissue trauma (see Chapter 10.6). Closed anatomical reduction of the fracture by traction and pressure is a prerequisite, but this cannot always be achieved. Often, this method can only provide reduction fixation (adaptive fixation).

10.4.1 Procedure

- A gliding hole with the same size as the screw diameter is drilled in the ipsilateral cortex, extending no further than the fracture gap (▶ Fig. 10.4a).
- Insert a drill guide (▶ Fig. 10.4b).
- Always drill the threaded hole through a guide: otherwise, axial deviations may occur in the threaded hole and these can lead to fracture of the cortex when the lag screw is tightened (▶ Fig. 10.4c).
- Drill a threaded hole in the contralateral cortex through the drill guide, with the diameter of the screw core (▶ Fig. 10.4d).
- Measure the screw lengths using a gage (▶ Fig. 10.4e).
- When measuring the screw length, measure the shorter length by rotating the hook on the gage. If the self-tapping screw is too long, soft tissue injury may occur, involving the flexor tendons, for example (▶ Fig. 10.4f).
- Introduce a self-tapping screw of the correct length and diameter (▶ Fig. 10.4g).

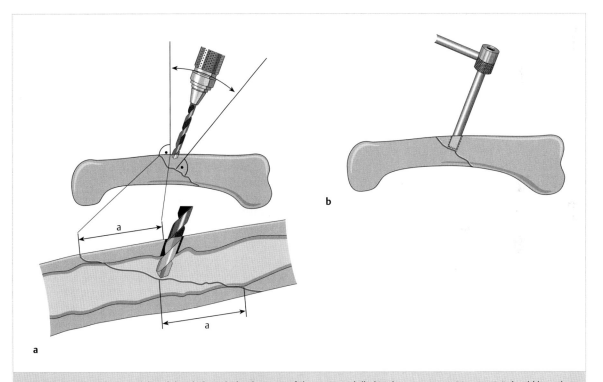

Fig. 10.4 Lag screw fixation. **(a)** A gliding hole with the diameter of the screw is drilled in the near cortex. Distance "a" should be as long as possible; see ▶ Fig. 10.5h; for the drilling direction, see ▶ Fig. 10.5d. **(b)** A drill guide is introduced into the gliding hole.

Continued ▶

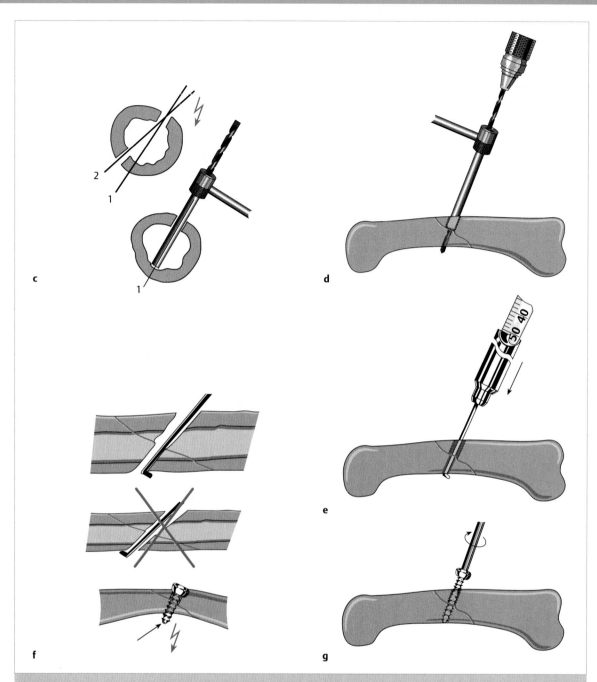

Fig. 10.4 *(Continued)* **(c)** The threaded hole should always be drilled only through the drill guide in the gliding hole. If drilling is not guided (1), axial deviation can occur in the threaded hole (2), which may result in fracture of the cortex when the lag screw is tightened. See also ▶ Fig. 10.5h. **(d)** Drill a threaded hole with the diameter of the screw core through the far cortex. See ▶ Fig. 10.5h. **(e)** Measure the screw length with a gage. **(f)** Measure the shorter screw length by rotating the hook of the gage; otherwise, the inserted screw will project beyond the far cortex with a risk of soft tissue damage, e.g., flexor tendon injury. **(g)** Introduce a self-tapping lag screw. See ▶ Fig. 10.5h.

Practical Tips

- If a Kirschner wire was inserted for temporary fracture fixation, this must be removed before the screw is finally tightened to produce interfragmental compression so that locking is avoided.
- If there is a risk for the screw head to sink in (e.g., because of poor cortical quality or in the metaphyseal region), use a washer (▸ Fig. 10.5a).
- When using small-diameter screws, drill only the ipsilateral cortex to obtain adequate purchase over a longer part of the small thread (▸ Fig. 10.5b).
- Whenever possible, drill and insert the screw from the smaller fragment to the bigger one (▸ Fig. 10.5c).
- The optimal angle for the lag screw is one half of the angle between the cortex and fracture line (▸ Fig. 10.5d).

- On transverse section through the bone, the lag screws should be as far as possible perpendicular to the fracture plane (▸ Fig. 10.5e).
- Several screws of smaller diameter achieve better compression and greater stability than one screw with a larger diameter (▸ Fig. 10.5f).
- If the lag screw is located in the area covered by the plate because of the course of the fracture, pass the lag screw through the plate (▸ Fig. 10.5g).
- Ensure that the hole is drilled at a sufficient distance from the apex of the fracture. Otherwise there is a risk of longitudinal fracture of the tip of the fragment when a gliding hole is drilled and when compression is produced by the lag screw (▸ Fig. 10.5h).

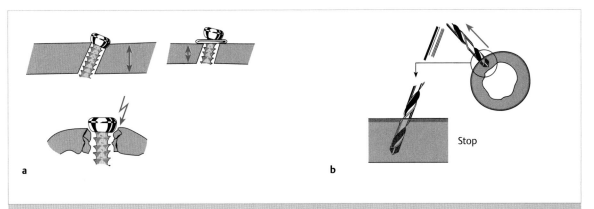

a   b

Fig. 10.5 Tips for lag screw fixation. **(a)** If the cortex is damaged and fragile, e.g., because of osteoporosis, and in the metaphyseal region, use a washer to prevent collapse of the lag screw. **(b)** When using a thin screw diameter, drill only the near cortex so as to achieve better traction of the lag screw.

Continued ▸

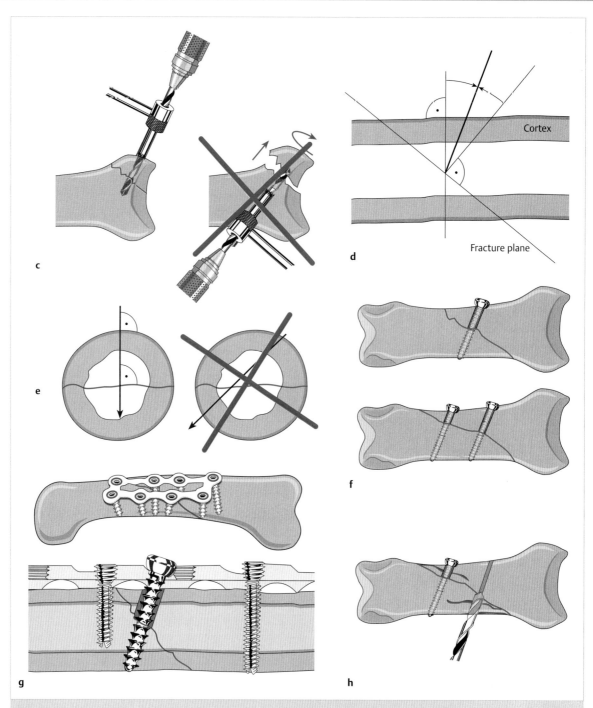

Fig. 10.5 *(Continued)* **(c)** When drilling a small fracture fragment, always drill from the smaller to the larger fragment. Otherwise there is a risk that drilling will cause dislocation. **(d)** The ideal direction for drilling is one-half of the angle between a perpendicular to the fracture plane and a perpendicular to the plane of the cortex. € Whenever possible, drill perpendicularly to the fracture plane and avoid acute angles, especially to the fracture plane. **(f)** Interfragmental compression is safer and provides greater stability if two lag screws of smaller diameter are used rather than one lag screw of greater diameter. **(g)** Depending on the course of the fracture, a lag screw can also pass through a plate. The other screws in the plate can be fixed-angle locking and standard cortical types. **(h)** When the ends of the fracture are tapered, there is a risk of longitudinal fracture due to drilling of a gliding hole or compression of the lag screw.

10.5 Lag Screw plus Neutralization Plate

10.5.1 Procedure

- Insert a lag screw to produce interfragmental compression (▶ Fig. 10.6a; see Chapter 10.4.1).
- Match the shape of the plate (size and design) to the anatomy and place it in position.
- Place a standard cortical screw in the proximal plate hole, especially when using T- and L-plates (drill, measure, insert the screw). Before fully tightening the screw, align the axis of the plate correctly with the shaft of the bone (▶ Fig. 10.6b).
- Only then, place the second screw in the short limb of the plate (▶ Fig. 10.6c).
- Place screws in the remaining plate holes; fixed-angle locking screws may be used for better stability (▶ Fig. 10.6d).

- Drilling for screws in the head of H-, L-, and T-plates should diverge from proximal to distal to avoid the screws colliding intraosseously (▶ Fig. 10.6e).

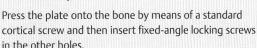

Practical Tip

Press the plate onto the bone by means of a standard cortical screw and then insert fixed-angle locking screws in the other holes.

Practical tip

If the plate is fixed exclusively with fixed-angle locking screws, it must be contoured and placed exactly anatomically as otherwise there is a risk of too great a gap between plate and bone.

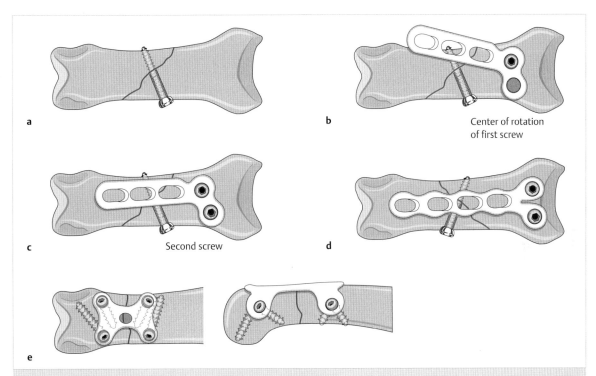

a

b   Center of rotation of first screw

c   Second screw

d

e

Fig. 10.6 Lag screw plus neutralization plate. **(a)** The fracture is first fixed with a lag screw to generate interfragmental compression in the gap (see Chapter 10.4.1 and note Fig. 10.5h). As sufficient stability from this measure cannot be expected, a plate is applied in addition, which neutralizes the forces acting from without (neutralization plate). **(b)** When an L-shaped plate is used for neutralization, it is first shaped anatomically. A standard cortical screw is placed in the hole in the long axis. The plate is aligned correctly with the shaft before it is finally tightened. **(c)** After fixing the plate to the bone in the correct axis, a screw is placed in the second hole of the short limb. This ensures the longitudinal alignment of the plate. **(d)** Fixed-angle locking screws can be placed in the remaining holes to provide what is known as a hybrid plate. **(e)** When H-, L-, or T-plates are used, it must be ensured that the positions of the screws diverge to avoid screw collisions.

10.6 Percutaneous Lag Screw

Percutaneous lag screw fixation has become established in line with minimization of operation trauma and technical developments. It can be used for
• juxta-articular fractures and
• spiral and oblique phalangeal fractures.

▶ **Prerequisites and advantages.** A special instrument—the lag screw target bow / reduction forceps—for lag screws, is required. The fracture is reduced and fixed with this multifunctional instrument under image intensification, percutaneously or subcutaneously (using a different target bow). At the same time, this special reduction instrument acts as a drill guide and gage for measuring lag screw length (▶ Fig. 10.7).

The advantage is the minimally invasive approach, which leads to less soft tissue damage. This method is a sophisticated technique that requires experience. It must be possible to reduce the fracture exactly; both reduction and fixation are possible only under image intensifier control.

If adequate compression of the fracture is achieved with the multifunctional instrument, it may be possible to replace the typical lag screw by a fixation screw or screws, thereby reducing the risk of a longitudinal fracture (see also ▶ Fig. 10.5h).

10.6.1 Procedure

• The incision is followed by minimal soft tissue dissection at the level of the fracture.
• The appropriate target bow / reduction forceps for the lag screw to be used (percutaneous or subcutaneous) is placed on either side of the fracture.
• The toothed end of the lag screw target bow is placed directly on the bone through the minimally invasive tissue opening according to the line of the fracture.
• Interfragmental compression and fixation of the fracture are obtained by closing the multifunctional instrument (▶ Fig. 10.8a).
• X-rays are taken in two planes and rotation is checked by flexing the fingers.
• The appropriate drill guide is introduced, initially with the diameter of the screw core.
• Drill through both cortices (▶ Fig. 10.8a).
• Exchange the drill and its guide for drilling the gliding hole (lag screw diameter).
• Drill a gliding hole in the near cortex through the appropriate new drill guide (▶ Fig. 10.8b) and measure the length.
• Insert the screw guide sleeve.
• Screw in the self-tapping lag screw (▶ Fig. 10.8c).
• Repeat this procedure if a second lag screw is placed (long oblique fracture / spiral fracture) (▶ Fig. 10.8d).
• Remove the lag screw target bow and suture the skin.
• An alternative technique, after closing the multifunctional instrument and taking a check X-ray, is to introduce a guide wire and place a self-tapping headless bone screw / cannulated fixation screw of appropriate length.

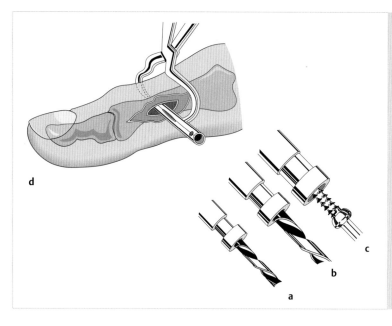

Fig. 10.7 Lag screw target bow/reduction forceps devices are all based on the same principle, with drill guides and screw guide sleeves that can be exchanged. The lag screw target bow can be placed beyond the fracture, both percutaneously or after exposure of the bone. **(a)** Drill guide for screw core diameter (fixation hole). **(b)** Drill guide for screw diameter (gliding hole). **(c)** Screw guide sleeve. **(d)** Percutaneous application of the target bow/reduction forceps on the other side of the fracture.

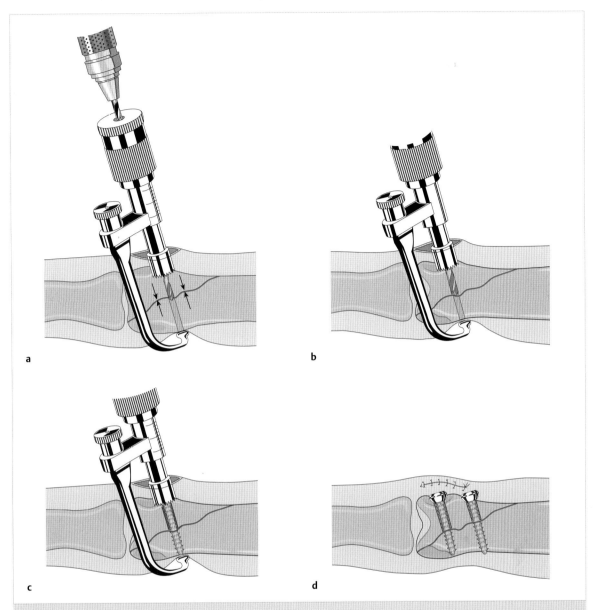

Fig. 10.8 Percutaneous lag screw fixation. **(a)** Following incision, the soft tissues are dissected bluntly, the bone is exposed minimally, and the lag screw target bow/reduction forceps device is applied. The fracture is reduced under X-ray control and the fracture is compressed by closing the multifunctional instrument. A fixation hole is first drilled through both cortices with the drill guide for the screw core diameter. **(b)** The drill guide is exchanged for the gliding hole (screw diameter) and the gliding hole is drilled as far as the fracture gap. **(c)** The screw length is determined by a gage and a self-tapping standard cortical screw is inserted using the screw guide sleeve. **(d)** In long oblique or spiral fractures, two lag screws can also be inserted.

10.7 Plate Fixation

Various materials and principles are possible when plates are used for internal fixation. At least stable fixation of the fracture is usually achieved. Commonly used plates include:
- Standard/classic plates
- Condylar plates
- Dynamic compression plates
- Fixed-angle locking plates—internal fixator
- Hybrid plates

▶ **Holes.** Plates with holes suitable exclusively for standard cortical screws are supplied by the industry:
- Rotation hole
- Compression hole
- Oval compression hole

In addition, there are plates with holes that accept both standard cortical screws and locking screws:
- Locking hole
- Combination hole
- Round hole

▶ **Standard/classic plates.** The stability of a fracture that is managed by fixation with a standard plate and standard cortical screws is produced by the friction between the underside of the plate and the surface of the bone. This requires that the screws be placed firmly in the bone, which is usually ensured by screwing them through both cortices. The disadvantage is that the compression between plate and bone interferes with periosteal perfusion.

Internal fixation with a condylar plate is based on the same principle. Their use is limited to the metaphyses of the fingers.

▶ **Locking plates.** See Chapter 10.8.

▶ **Hybrid plates.** Plates with locking holes or combination holes can be fixed both with standard cortical screws and with fixed-angle locking screws. When these plates are combined with the two types of screws, they are called hybrid plates (hybrid screw construct).

This type of fixation is preferred for metaphyseal and epiphyseal fractures. The standard cortical screw generally acts as an interfragmental compression or lag screw to restore a smooth joint surface in the case of intra-articular fractures. Fixed-angle locking screws are placed in the shaft to provide axial and rotational stability.

10.7.1 Interfragmental Compression

The stability of plate fixation can be increased by interfragmental compression. However, interfragmental compression with a plate can only be achieved in a few extra-articular fractures of the shaft.
- Transverse fractures
- Short oblique fractures

Interfragmental compression by means of a lag screw (or screws) is possible in:
- Avulsion fractures
- Long oblique fractures
- Certain intra-articular mono- and bicondylar fractures

There are different methods of achieving interfragmental compression in the region of a fracture (or osteotomy) with a plate:
- Dynamic axial compression by eccentric drilling (spherical gliding principle)
- By tension device
- By central bending of the plate

Interfragmental Compression According to the Spherical Gliding Principle

By drilling eccentrically in an oval plate hole away from the fracture (or less often in a round hole), a thrust on the plate is created when the standard cortical screw is tightened, due to the round shape of the underside of the screw head. The bone fragment is pressed against the opposite side in the region of the fracture. The interplay of the screw hole shape and the eccentric placement of the screw in the hole of the plate creates axial compression.
- Select a plate of size and design appropriate to the anatomy and fracture type.
- Place a plate with oval holes (combination holes), shaped to match the anatomy as precisely as possible, on the bone, usually on the tension band side.
- Carefully reduce the fracture, ensuring correct rotation and axes in both planes.
- Fix the plate *close to the fracture* with a standard cortical screw and neutral, noneccentric drilling: drill, measure screw length, and insert the screw (▶ Fig. 10.9a), firstly, if possible, in the fragment nearer to the joint
- Then drill eccentrically *away from the fracture* in the hole next to the fracture in the further-away fragment opposite the already fixed fragment: measure the screw length and insert a standard cortical screw (▶ Fig. 10.9b).

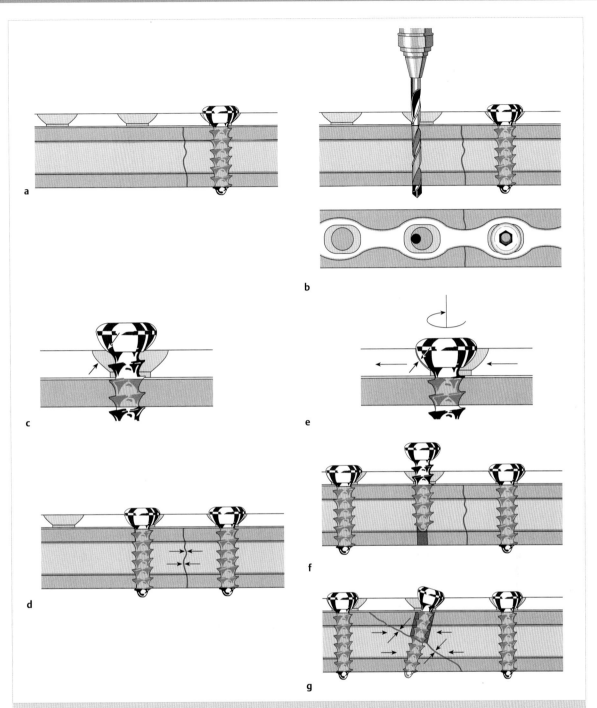

Fig. 10.9 Interfragmental compression using the spherical gliding principle. **(a)** To obtain compression of the fracture by means of the spherical gliding principle, the plate must first be secured through a hole close to the fracture by neutral drilling and standard cortical screw fixation. **(b)** Drill non-neutrally and asymmetrically in the plate hole away from the fracture, i.e., in the oval compression hole, at the side of the hole further away from the fracture. **(c)** When the standard cortical screw is tightened, the rounded underside of the screw head collides with the "lopsided" underside of the plate hole. **(d)** When it is tightened further, the plate moves on the bone surface and the screw head slips into the neutral position of the plate hole. **(e)** This interplay produces compression of the fracture. **(f)** Increased fracture compression can be achieved by double use of the spherical gliding principle but the already-placed second screw must be loosened somewhat before the third screw, placed the other side of the fracture, is finally tightened. **(g)** With oblique fractures, the interfragmental compression can be increased or stabilized by an additional lag screw.

- When the screw is tightened, the fragment will be pushed toward the fracture site. This generates axial compression on the fracture (▶ Fig. 10.9c, ▶ Fig. 10.9d, ▶ Fig. 10.9e).
- Compression can be increased by placing a second supplementary screw eccentrically in the adjacent hole (▶ Fig. 10.9f).

Practical Tip

Before finally tightening the third screw, the second screw must be loosened a little (▶ Fig. 10.9f). The stability of the screw core must not be strained when it is tightened (because of the risk of the screw head breaking).

- Then place cortical screws or fixed-angle locking screws in the other holes of the plate, as necessary.
- In the case of oblique fractures, interfragmental compression can be further increased by a lag screw introduced through the plate (▶ Fig. 10.9g).

Practical Tips

To avoid axial deviation and rotation errors when T- and L-plates are used, the following should be noted:
- The plate must be curved exactly to fit the anatomy of the bone.
- Drill the first hole in the smaller fragment in the long axis of the bone shaft (▶ Fig. 10.10a).

- Fix the plate with the first screw in the smaller fragment (▶ Fig. 10.10a).
- Reduce the longer fragment in the correct axis and check the rotation. Fix it temporarily with a plate reduction forceps (▶ Fig. 10.10a).
- If necessary, correct the reduction by bending, rotating, or twisting the plate.
- Place the second screw in the smaller fragment (▶ Fig. 10.10b).
- Again check the axis and rotation and correct if necessary by bending, rotating, or twisting the plate.
- Drill in the larger fragment eccentrically, as described above (▶ Fig. 10.10c).
- Tighten the screw to obtain interfragmental compression (▶ Fig. 10.10d).
- Only when the plate is placed correctly and the fracture is in anatomical position, place cortical screws or fixed-angle locking screws in the rest of the holes in the larger fragment.

Interfragmental Compression by Tension Device

- Select a plate of size and design appropriate to the fracture type.
- Contour and adjust it to the anatomy.
- Reduce the fracture exactly, ensuring correct rotation and axes in both planes.

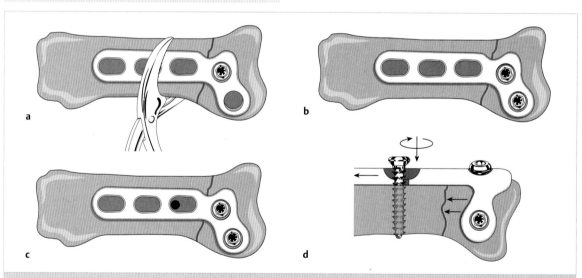

Fig. 10.10 Avoidance of axial deviation and rotation errors during interfragmental compression according to the spherical gliding principle.
(a) For fractures in the metaphyseal region, the L- or T-plates must first be fixed in the smaller fragment next to the joint with a neutrally drilled screw in the long axis of the bigger shaft fragment. After aligning the plate in the correct axis, rotation is checked and the bigger fragment is fixed temporarily with the plate using a reduction forceps.
(b) The second plate hole in the smaller fragment next to the joint is also fixed neutrally with a diverging screw.
(c) As described above (▶ Fig. 10.9b), an asymmetric hole is drilled away from the fracture (view from above).
(d) Fracture compression is produced by tightening the screw (see ▶ Fig. 10.9e) (lateral view).

- Fix the plate close to the fracture, if possible on the tension band side and, if possible, in the smaller fragment, usually close to the joint.

> **Note**
>
> When fixed-angle locking screws or a fixed-angle locking plate is used, the plate must be contoured precisely to the anatomy.

- Check before placing the second screw:
  - Is the plate lying exactly on the bone?
  - Is there any rotational error?
- Place the second screw in the smaller fragment, usually the one closer to the joint; in this way, the plate is stabilized in the fragment with the rotation and axis correct (► Fig. 10.11a); usually it is not necessary to use fixed-angle locking screws in the smaller metaphyseal fragment.
- The anatomically reduced fracture is fixed temporarily using a plate reduction forceps:
  - A hole is drilled through the cortex outside and in extension of the plate, large enough for one pointed jaw of a reduction forceps to be seated securely; the hole must be drilled at a slight angle from dorsal further from the plate to palmar closer to the plate.
  - The second jaw of the reduction forceps is inserted in one of the holes of the plate already fixed (► Fig. 10.11b).
- Interfragmental compression is produced by closing the reduction forceps (► Fig. 10.11c).
- After checking the axis and rotation, screws are inserted in the free holes, using standard cortical screws or fixed-angle locking screws

> **Note**
>
> Insert the screws in diverging direction to avoid intraosseous screw collision (► Fig. 10.11d)!

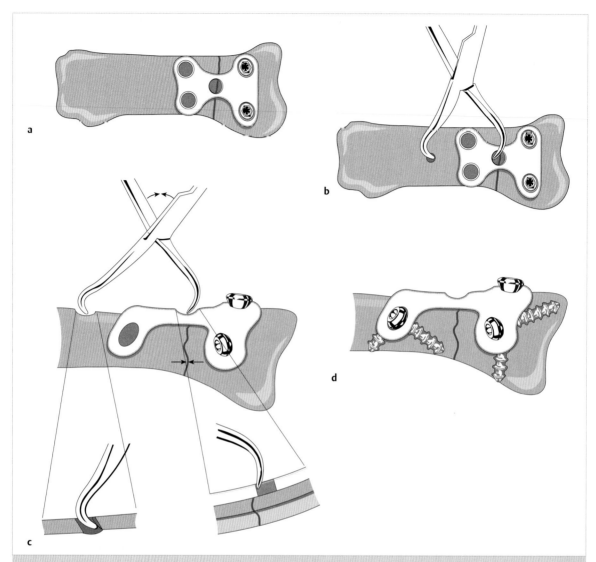

Fig. 10.11 Interfragmental compression with an tension device. **(a)** The plate is fixed neutrally, usually in the smaller fragment first. When L-, T- or H-plates are used, the fracture is reduced anatomically and rotation checked. A neutral screw is placed in the smaller fragment in the second plate hole. If fixed-angle locking screws are used, the plate must fit the bone very precisely. **(b)** A hole is drilled outside the plate in the long axis of the plate obliquely angled toward the plate. The diameter must admit one pointed jaw of a reduction forceps. The other jaw of the reduction forceps is inserted in a plate hole of the already-fixed plate. **(c)** The fragment is compressed by closing the forceps. **(d)** After checking the axis and rotation, screws are inserted in the remaining plate holes to maintain interfragmental compression, ensuring that the screws are in diverging positions.

Interfragmental Compression by Bending the Center of the Plate

This procedure should be regarded only as a reserve measure, as it has not been proven effective when plates are used in the hand. It can be employed only with standard cortical screws.

- The plate is bent beforehand so that the ends sit on the bone and there is a gap between the plate and the bone at the level of the fracture.
- The plate is first fixed at the two outer holes (▶ Fig. 10.12a).
- The other holes are then filled from outward to the center, alternating the two sides (▶ Fig. 10.12b).
- Compression in the fracture region is produced by pushing the fragments toward each other, "pulling" the bone toward the plate (▶ Fig. 10.12c).

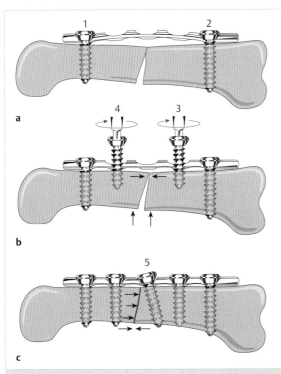

Fig. 10.12 Interfragmental compression by prior bending of the center of the plate. This method has not become accepted in the hand. It should only be used as an alternative in an emergency. It can be done only with standard cortical screws. **(a)** The ends of a plate bent in the center are fixed. **(b)** The free holes are then filled, moving from the outer ends to the center, alternating the two sides. **(c)** Final appearance with compression of the fracture.

10.8 Fixed-Angle Locking Plate—Internal Fixator

10.8.1 Principles

The unidirectional locking screw requires that drilling through the plate hole and bone is in a precisely defined direction. The locking screws can be inserted in a multi-axial drill-guide funnel of ± 10° or 20° depending on the manufacturer (see Chapter 8.2).

As regards stability, internal fixation of a fracture with a plate and locking screws represents an internal fixator. The plate and screws form a stable, rigid unit that is independent of friction between the plate and bone surface and depends mainly on the rigidity of the construction.

Fixation of a fracture with controlled minimal movement in the fracture region is important for fracture healing. Complete rigid fixation without interfragmental compression must be avoided as it leads more often to delayed bone union or even pseudarthrosis. The axis, rotation, and length of the bone should be restored by reduction; in the case of intra-articular fractures, a completely stable joint surface without step-off must be achieved first by interfragmental compression using lag screws.

Bridging fixed-angle locking plates can be used for osteoporotic bone and extensive areas of comminution. In these situations the fixed-angle locking operation technique represents major progress (▶ Fig. 10.13).

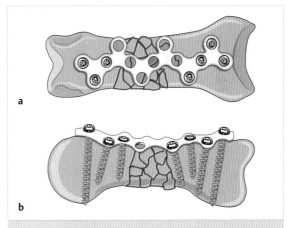

Fig. 10.13 Management of a shaft fracture with an extensive comminution zone using fixed-angle locking fixation by means of a bridging plate, e.g., using a staggered Z-plate. **(a)** View from above. **(b)** Lateral view.

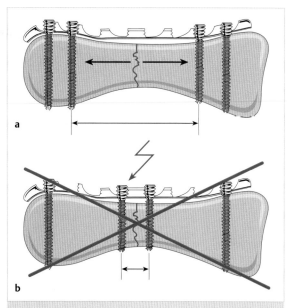

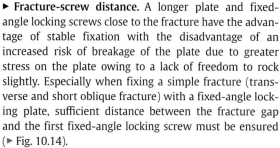

Fig. 10.14 Fixed-angle locking of simple fractures. **(a)** With simple fractures (transverse and short oblique shaft fractures), sufficient distance between the fracture gap and the fixed-angle locking screw fixation must be ensured. **(b)** If the distance is too small, there is a risk of plate fracture due to increased stress on the plate.

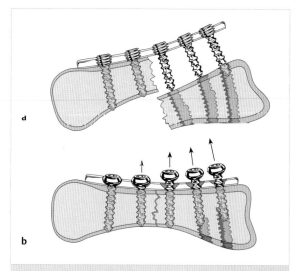

Fig. 10.15 Loosening of a fixed-angle locking plate. **(a)** When the rigid internal fixator construction is used, loosening always involves the entire construction. **(b)** When standard cortical screws are used for fixation, screw loosening is linear.

▶ **Fracture-screw distance.** A longer plate and fixed-angle locking screws close to the fracture have the advantage of stable fixation with the disadvantage of an increased risk of breakage of the plate due to greater stress on the plate owing to a lack of freedom to rock slightly. Especially when fixing a simple fracture (transverse and short oblique fracture) with a fixed-angle locking plate, sufficient distance between the fracture gap and the first fixed-angle locking screw must be ensured (▶ Fig. 10.14).

Based on experience with large bones, the following applies theoretically for the bones of the fingers:
- The plate length should be at least three times as long as the comminution zone.
- Not more than 50% of the plate holes should be occupied.
- Fixed-angle locking screws should be inserted in at least three holes in each main fragment, and in osteoporotic bone these should always be bicortical.
- The closer the third fixed-angle locking screw is to the fracture, the more rigid the construction.
- The greater the distance between the plate and the bone surface, the lower the stability.

▶ **Loosening.** When a fixed-angle locking fixation becomes mechanically loose, the construction always

becomes loosened from the bone as a whole (▶ Fig. 10.15a). Occasionally, a single fixed-angle locking screw may loosen when the plate hole is deformed with multiaxial screws, leading to loss of fixed-angle locking. When the plate is fixed with standard cortical screws, screw loosening is usually linear (▶ Fig. 10.15b).

▶ **Suitable plates..** Because of the anatomy of the hand and fingers, especially the relatively short length of the digital bones, the possibilities for using simple, linear fixed-angle locking plates are limited. 3D, grid, mesh, trapeze, and Z-plates may be useful as they provide space for several fixed-angle locking screws with a shorter length (▶ Fig. 10.16). Hybrid plates, which allow combined use of standard screws and fixed-angle locking screws for plate fixation, may also be used (hybrid screw construct).

> **Note**
>
> The most stable construction with the best potential for primary bone healing consists of interfragmental lag screw compression independent of a plate, combined with a fixed-angle locking plate (▶ Fig. 10.17).

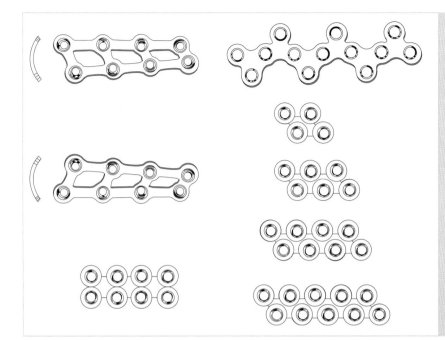

Fig. 10.16 To avoid stress on the plate by having the fixed-angle locking screws at sufficient distance, use of multidimensional plates is highly recommended.

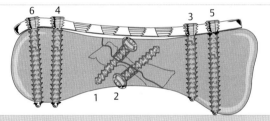

Fig. 10.17 Deliberate combined use of standard cortical screws and fixed-angle locking screws is always possible. The most stable treatment consists of fixation with lag screws independent of a plate (1, 2), combined with a fixed-angle locking plate (3–6).

10.8.2 Procedure

- Ensure that the plate and screws are the same size, usually by means of color coding.
- Adapt an implant of suitable design and size to the anatomy (▶ Fig. 10.18a).
- Screw the appropriate unidirectional drill guide into the plate (▶ Fig. 10.18b).
- Drill in the given direction through the guide in the near cortex and, if necessary, also through the far cortex (▶ Fig. 10.18c).
- Determine the screw length with a gage.
- Insert the screw and tighten it cautiously in the plate (▶ Fig. 10.18d).

Caution

When tightening the screw there is a danger of deforming the thread and removal of the implant will then no longer be possible.

Note

- ○ A plate should only be bent between the holes so as not to deform the threaded holes when bending the plate; otherwise the plate and the screw head will be incongruent (▶ Fig. 10.19a, b).
- ○ A better method is to place bending pins or drill guides or long fixed-angle locking screws loosely in the holes so that the plate can then be bent correctly (▶ Fig. 10.19c, d).

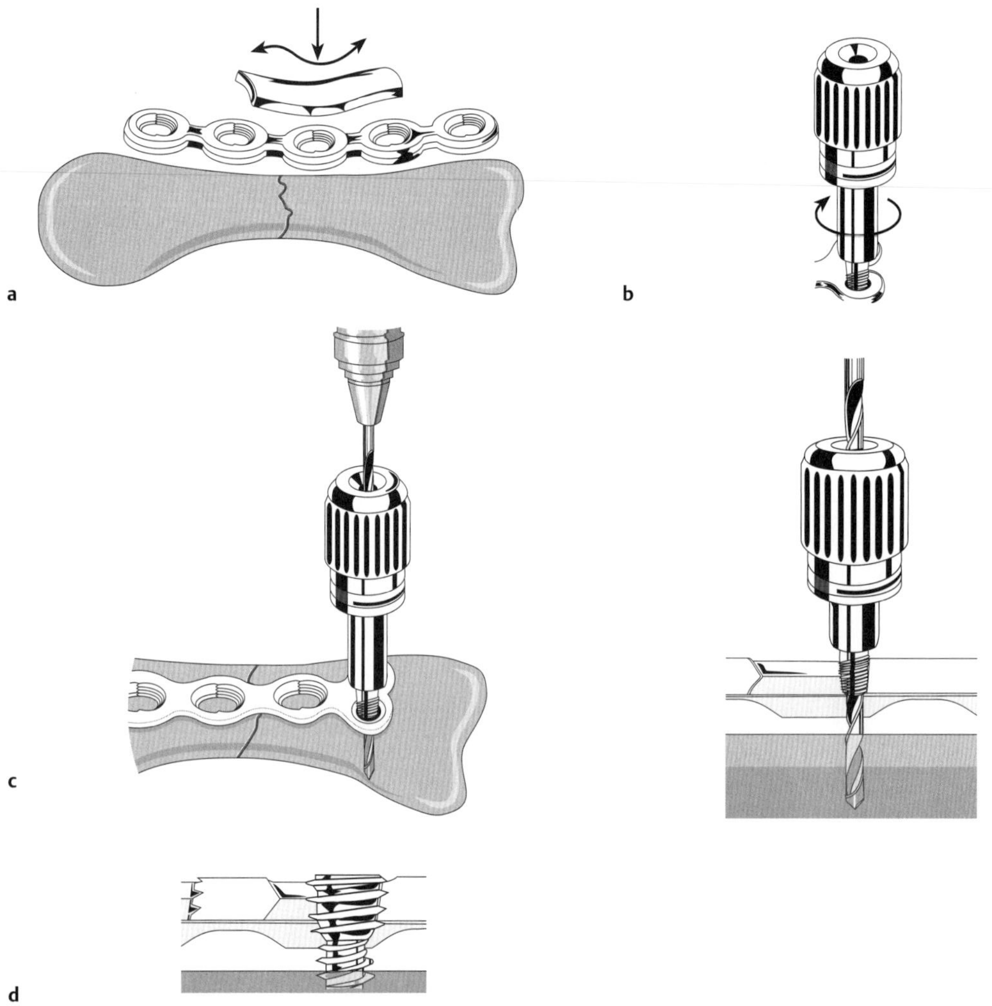

Fig. 10.18 Internal fixator. **(a)** When a fixed-angle locking plate is used, it must be ensured that the size and design of the plate match the anatomy of the bone as precisely as possible before it is fixed (note color coding). They should fit together in all planes to keep the distance between bone and plate as small as possible. This increases the stability of the internal fixation. **(b)** After the plate is placed on the bone, the unidirectional drill guide is screwed on. **(c)** Drill with the screw core diameter in the predetermined direction in the near cortex and, if necessary, in the far cortex. **(d)** Fix the fixed-angle locking screw of correct size (note color coding) carefully in the thread of the plate.

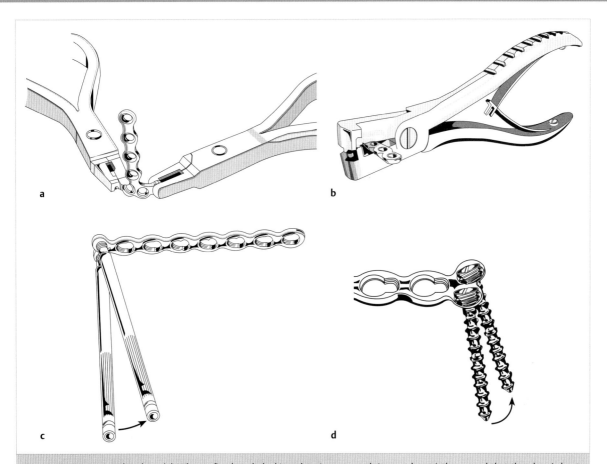

Fig. 10.19 Contouring the plate. **(a)** When a fixed-angle locking plate is contoured, it must be strictly ensured that the plate is bent between the holes to avoid incongruence between the thread of the plate and the thread of the screw head. Special bending devices are available. **(b)** Plate cutting tools are also available. **(c)** Use of bending pins is recommended. **(d)** An alternative possibility: Place long fixed-angle locking screws in the plate holes and contour the plate to the correct shape with the aid of the inserted screws.

▶ **Multidirectional system**

- When using a multidirectional system, ensure that the plate and screws are the same size, usually by means of color coding.
- Contour and adjust an implant of suitable design and size for the anatomy.
- Attach the multidirectional drill guide (▶ Fig. 10.20, ▶ Fig. 10.20b).
- Drill through the guide in the planned direction in the near cortex and, if necessary, in the far cortex also (▶ Fig. 10.20c).

- Determine the screw length with a gage (▶ Fig. 10.20d).
- Insert the screw in the plate and tighten it cautiously (▶ Fig. 10.20e).

> ⚠
> ### Caution
> When the screw is tightened, there is a risk of cold welding, whereby screw removal may become impossible.

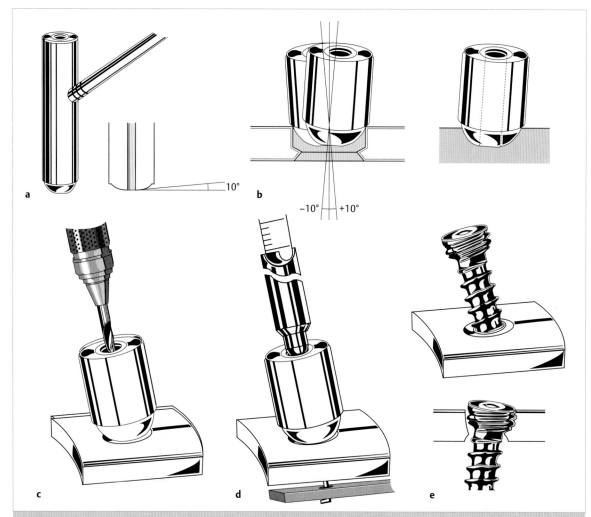

Fig. 10.20 Multidirectional system. **(a)** When multidirectional fixed-angle locking screws are used, the special guide for multidirectional drilling is attached, after adapting the plate precisely to the anatomy. A direction of ± 10° (20°) can be selected within a drill funnel. **(b)** Section through the attached drill guide. **(c)** Drilling in the planned direction with the screw core diameter. **(d)** When measuring screw length, select the shorter length, either by rotating the gage (as shown here; see also ▶ Fig. 10.4f) or by reading it from the scale. **(e)** Screw the multidirectional fixed-angle locking screw carefully in the thread of the plate. There is a danger of cold welding, which can render later implant removal very difficult or impossible. There is also a risk of breakage of the screw head.

10.9 Condylar Plate

Condylar plates are used mainly for **T**- and **Y**-shaped fractures that are intra-articular or extra-articular but close to a joint.

10.9.1 Procedure

- With intra-articular fractures, the joint is opened, the fracture is reduced without step-off and fixed temporarily by a Kirschner wire parallel to the joint surface (▶ Fig. 10.21a), or by means of a fine-pointed reduction forceps (▶ Fig. 10.21b).
- With an extra-articular fracture, a fine Kirschner wire is advanced through the joint, parallel to the joint surface. This is checked with the image intensifier (▶ Fig. 10.21c).
- When a Kirschner wire is used for temporary fixation, the wire must be placed in such a way that it can be replaced by a screw or lag screw after the condylar plate is applied, that is, dorsal or palmar to the shaft axis (▶ Fig. 10.21d).
- Advance the drill guide over the Kirschner wire and place it on the fragment at an angle of 90° to the shaft axis (▶ Fig. 10.21e).
- Drill parallel to the Kirschner wire, that is, parallel to the joint surface, through the condyles. The hole diameter must be big enough to take the condylar blade or a fixed-angle buttress pin (Fig. 10.21f); the fixed-angle buttress pin corresponds to the condylar blade.
- Measure the length of the blade or fixed-angle buttress pin.
- Introduce the blade of the condylar plate or a buttress pin attached to the plate provisionally into the predrilled channel (▶ Fig. 10.21g).

- The plate must now sit exactly on the bone. Check its position on the shaft and check rotation and contour the plate appropriately.

> **Caution**
>
> There is a risk of fracturing the fragment when the plate is screwed into place.

- When contouring is topographically exact, the condylar plate or plate with fixed-angle buttress pin is finally inserted (▶ Fig. 10.21h).
- The Kirschner wire is removed after securing the fracture with pointed reduction forceps and the plate is fixed to the bone shaft (▶ Fig. 10.21i).
- For a T- or Y-shaped fracture, place a lag screw, if possible, in the proximal plate hole next to the head. A lag screw may also be placed in the distal fragment (▶ Fig. 10.21j).
- The plate is fixed to the shaft by a cortical screw, if possible with dynamic compression (see Chapter 10.7.1) and/or a fixed-angle locking screw (▶ Fig. 10.21k); use a lag screw for an oblique metaphyseal fracture (▶ Fig. 10.21l).

> **Note**
>
> This is a difficult internal fixation technique as there is a risk of condylar fracture by the blade. The bone fragment bearing the condylar blade or buttress pin must always be fixed with an additional screw.

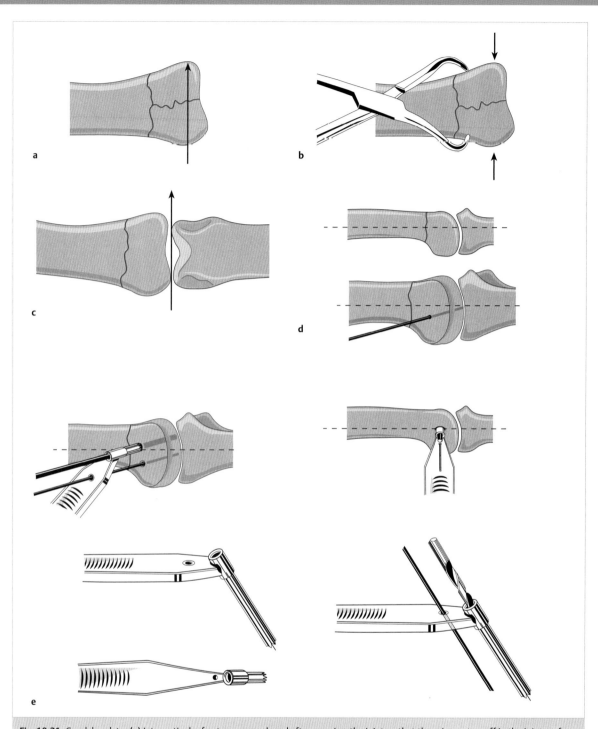

Fig. 10.21 Condylar plate. **(a)** Intra-articular fractures are reduced after opening the joint so that there is no step-off in the joint surface. They are then fixed temporarily with a Kirschner wire. **(b)** Alternatively, the fracture can be fixed with a pointed reduction forceps, with simultaneous interfragmental compression. **(c)** In the case of extra-articular metaphyseal fractures, a fine Kirschner wire is advanced for guidance through the joint under image intensifier control, parallel to the joint surface. **(d)** The intraosseous transverse Kirschner wire **(a)** should be placed in such a way that it can be replaced by a screw; ideally by a lag screw after the condylar plate is applied **(i, j)**. **(e)** The special drill guide is attached over the Kirschner wire. It must be ensured that the drill hole is in the long axis of the bone.

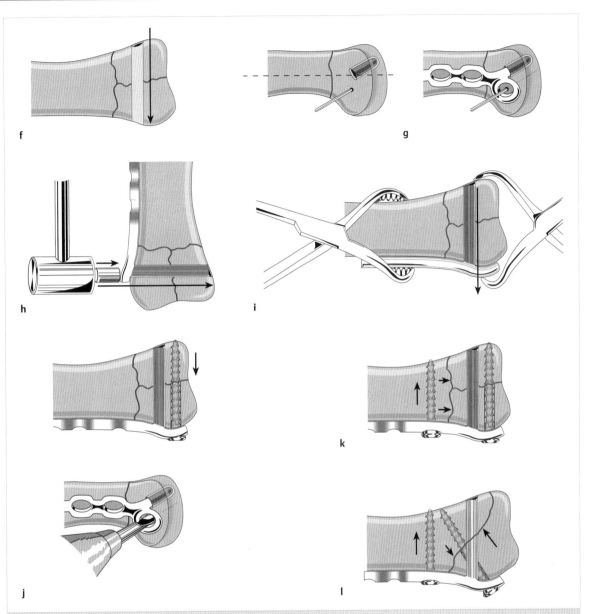

Fig. 10.21 (*Continued*) **(f)** Drilling with the screw core diameter. **(g)** After determining the length of the drill hole to accept the blade or buttress pin, the blade or pin is inserted temporarily in the previously drilled channel. **(h)** The condylar plate must now sit precisely on the bone surface, so appropriate contouring is extremely important. It is essential to align the plate along the long axis of the bone when the rotation and axis of the fracture has been fully corrected. The condylar blade or fixed-angle buttress pin is then finally inserted. **(i)** The condylar plate is fixed temporarily to the shaft using a plate reduction forceps. The intra-articular fracture is held with a pointed reduction forceps and the Kirschner wire is removed. **(j)** A hole of screw core diameter is drilled in the proximal plate on either side of the fracture. With T and Y shaped fractures, drill a gliding hole as far as the fracture if possible so that a lag screw can be placed. **(k)** The condylar plate is fixed to the shaft with standard cortical screws, as far as possible achieving interfragmental compression by asymmetric drilling away from the fracture (see Chapter 10.7.1). Fixed-angle locking is also possible. **(l)** With oblique metaphyseal fractures, compression of the fracture can also be obtained by a lag screw through the proximal plate hole.

10.10 Intraosseous Compression Screw, Headless Bone Screw, and Compression Wire

10.10.1 Principle and Indications

The intraosseous compression screw developed by Timothy Herbert has proved to be very effective for certain indications. Different versions are now commercially available, all based on the same principle.

Intraosseous compression screws are cannulated screws with a self-tapping thread at both ends; they come in different diameters, lengths, and thread pitches (▶ Fig. 10.22a). A modification of the screw developed by Herbert is a cannulated, headless, self-tapping screw. Gradual compression is obtained with each turn according to the varying design of the thread pitches (▶ Fig. 10.22b). The intraosseous compression wire is based on the same principle (▶ Fig. 10.22c).

The screw is countersunk fully in the bone (▶ Fig. 10.23).

▶ **Indications.** Indications for use of an intraosseous compression screw in the hand:

- Scaphoid fractures—always for unstable scaphoid fractures

- Fractures of the other carpal bones
- Pseudarthrosis of the carpal bones
- Intra- and extra-articular fractures of small bones with bone fragments
- Avulsion fractures, fractures of processes
- Arthrodesis of the distal interphalangeal joint
- Long oblique or spiral fractures of the shaft of the phalanges and metacarpals

10.10.2 Procedure with Intraosseous Compression Screws

- The approach to the end of the bone through which the intraosseous compression screw is placed should be minimally traumatic.
- Carry out closed or open reduction of the fracture.
- Place the Kirschner wire guide sleeve directly on the bone end (▶ Fig. 10.24a).
- Alternatively, introduce a jig and, depending on the fracture, compress the fracture lightly using a noncannulated screw (▶ Fig. 10.24b); this has been replaced by the use of cannulated intraosseous compression screws.
- The guide wire is introduced under image intensifier control in both planes at a low speed. It must pass exactly longitudinally and centrally through both fragments as far as the cortex opposite the entry site but not beyond this (▶ Fig. 10.24c).

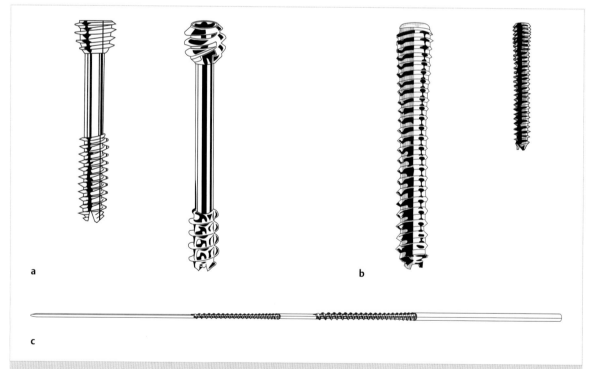

a

b

c

Fig. 10.22 Intraosseous compression screws and compression wire. **(a)** Cannulated intraosseous compression screws of different design. **(b)** One variant of the intraosseous compression screw is based on the same principle but with a different design. **(c)** Intraosseous compression wire.

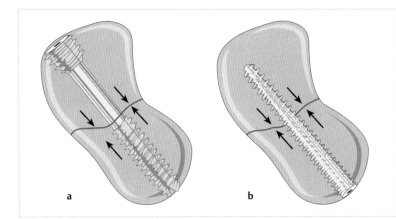

Fig. 10.23 (a,b) Compression screw, intraosseous. Principle: Fracture compression is achieved when the screw is tightened after crossing the fracture gap. The screws are available in different diameters, lengths, and thread pitches.

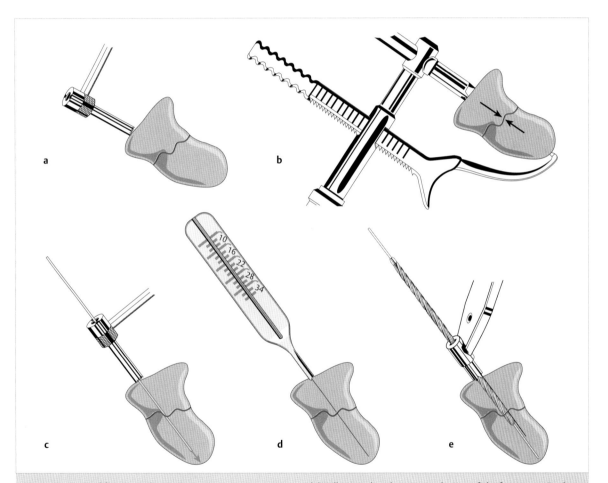

Fig. 10.24 Internal fixation with an intraosseous compression screw. (a) Following closed or open reduction of the fracture, a Kirschner wire guide sleeve is attached to the end of the bone in its long axis. (b) An alternative, but now out of fashion, is to attach a jig and obtain interfragmental compression using a noncannulated screw, depending on the course of the fracture. (c) Under image intensifier control and using a low drill speed, a Kirschner wire is introduced longitudinally in the exact center as far as the cortex beyond the fracture. (d) The screw length is measured on a scale. (e) Drill over the guide wire as far as the fracture gap or through the sclerosed pseudarthrosis or interposed bone graft using the correct drill size.

Continued ▶

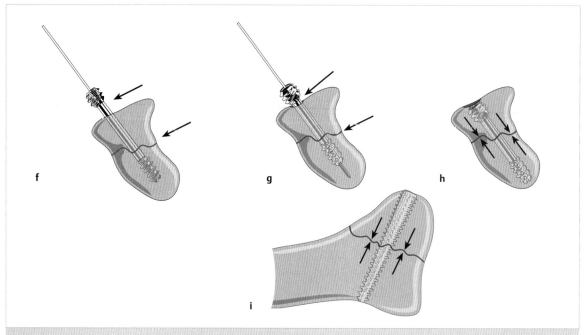

Fig. 10.24 *(Continued)* **(f)** Screw in the self-tapping headless bone screw over the guide wire until the distal thread has bridged the fracture gap, sclerosed pseudarthrosis, or interposed bone graft. **(g)** As soon as the distal thread has bridged the fracture gap, sclerosed pseudarthrosis, or interposed bone graft, remove the guide wire. The proximal thread must not yet touch the proximal end of the bone at this time. **(h)** The screw is inserted further until it is completely intraosseous. The distal end of the screw must still be intraosseous and must not perforate the distal cortex. **(i)** Edge fracture, shown as an example of using a different design of intraosseous compression screw.

- Determine the length with the gage for the intraosseous compression screw that is being used (▶ Fig. 10.24d).
- If the bone is sclerosed, drill a hole of appropriate diameter proximally as far as the fracture or to just beyond the pseudarthrosis (▶ Fig. 10.24e).
- Advance the intraosseous compression screw over the guide wire.
- Screw it in until the distal thread has bridged the fracture gap / pseudarthrosis / bone graft if the Herbert screw system was used (▶ Fig. 10.24f).

> **Note**
>
> The proximal thread on the near side must not touch the entry site on the bone until the distal thread has bridged the fracture gap, as only then is interfragmental compression obtained (Herbert screw system).

- As soon as the distal thread has bridged the fracture gap, remove the guide wire (▶ Fig. 10.24g), as otherwise

there is a risk of the cannulated screw and guide wire becoming jammed.
- Tighten the intraosseous compression screw fully until the proximal thread is countersunk slightly below the bone surface (▶ Fig. 10.24h, i).
- X-ray check in both planes and close the wound.

10.10.3 Procedure with the Percutaneous Compression Wire

- Make a short dorsoradial or dorsoulnar incision in the metaphyseal region of the proximal or middle phalanx.
- Expose the base of the phalanx using a blunt hemostat
- Following reduction of the fracture, predrill the compression wire percutaneously strictly outside the joint, under image intensifier control in both planes (▶ Fig. 10.25a, b)
- Drill through the cortex on the far side of the fracture.

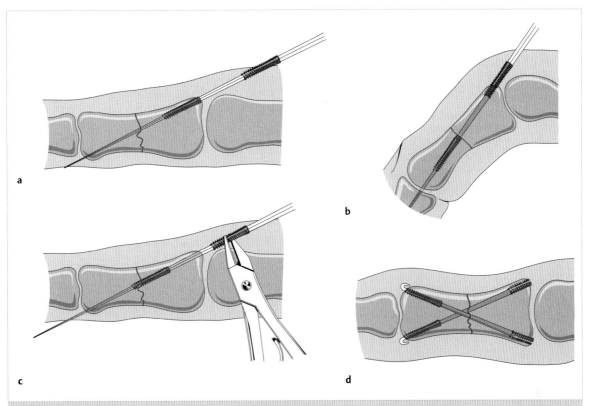

Fig. 10.25 Internal fixation with a percutaneous compression wire. **(a)** A stab skin incision is made, the base of the middle or proximal phalanx is exposed bluntly on the dorsoradial, and possibly also dorsoulnar, aspect. The wire is drilled until the tip is at the level of the fracture gap. Closed fracture reduction then takes place under image intensifier control in two planes. The wire is drilled further until it meets the opposite cortex, and the opposite cortex is then drilled through using a low drill speed and light pressure. View from above. **(b)** Lateral view. **(c)** Continue drilling until the tip of the wire threatens to perforate the skin. Make a stab incision over the tip of the wire. After advancing the wire, move the drill distally and drill antegradely until the proximal thread reaches skin level. The wire is nipped off, leaving 1 to 3 mm of the proximal thread. Under image intensifier control, continue antegrade drilling until the proximal thread just touches the base of the metaphysis. From this point, the wire is screwed in manually antegradely after bending the distal end to facilitate rotation. Once the proximal end is completely intraosseous, the distal end is shortened and bent so it can be buried subcutaneously. **(d)** For better stability, repeat the same procedure on the contralateral side.

 Caution

Use a low speed and low pressure because of the risk of the wire breaking and slipping.

- After drilling through the opposite cortex, continue drilling until skin perforation is imminent. As far as possible, avoid the lateral slips of the extensor tendon.
- Make an incision over the tip of the wire.
- Continue drilling the wire and move the drill distally to the tip of the wire, then advance the compression wire antegrade until the proximal thread has reached skin level.

- Cut off the proximal thread, leaving 1 to 3 mm of the thread.
- As soon as the proximal thread has reached the metaphyseal base of the bone under image intensifier control, bend the distal projecting wire and screw the compression wire in *manually* until the proximal thread is fully intraosseous (▶ Fig. 10.25c).
- After shortening the distal end, bend it and move the wire to a subcutaneous position.
- Carry out the same procedure on the contralateral side in order to achieve better stability (▶ Fig. 10.25d).
- Close the wound after intraoperative X-ray check.
- After fracture consolidation, the wire is removed antegrade.

10.11 Intramedullary Kirschner Wire Splinting or Pinning

Intramedullary Kirschner wire splinting or pinning has the advantage of access distant from the fracture. This means that the fracture hematoma is not affected. Secondary bone union through the hematoma, fibrous remodeling, and callus lead to surprisingly rapid bony fracture healing.

This is a minor procedure that is technically easy and associated with only minimal soft tissue damage. With this kind of fixation, protected early motion stability is usually successful. Only brief immobilization with a splint is necessary.

The method can be used retrogradely for proximal extra-articular fractures and antegradely for distal subcapital and shaft fractures of the middle and proximal phalanges, and especially for the metacarpal bones.

10.11.1 Procedure for Metacarpal Fractures

- Make a stab incision in the skin.
- Expose the entry portal for the pin or Kirschner wire by blunt dissection (▶ Fig. 10.26a).
- Open the metaphyseal medullary cavity with an awl or drill; do not perforate the opposite cortex (▶ Fig. 10.26b).
- Introduce a pin or Kirschner wire into the medullary cavity through a bone window.
- Advance a long drill sleeve over the pin or Kirschner wire to guide and stabilize it. This prevents the pin or wire from shifting while it is advanced.
- Bend the distal end of the pin or Kirschner wire slightly and bend the proximal end 90° in the same direction as the distal end; this allows a control of rotation even if the pin or Kirschner wire is already in intramedullary position (▶ Fig. 10.26c).
- Under image intensifier control, advance the intramedullary pin or wire.
- Advance it into the second fragment to obtain intramedullary bridging of the fracture gap.
- Advance the pin until it is in distal metaphyseal subchondral position. Compress the fracture (▶ Fig. 10.26d).
- Proceed in the same way with a second and possibly a third pin or Kirschner wire, advancing them antegrade in the metacarpal through the same opening (▶ Fig. 10.26e).

Practical Tip

Insert all other pins or Kirschner wires on the flexor side below the first insert as this enables it to provide better guidance for the others. If possible, place the pins or Kirschner wires like a bouquet of flowers in the contralateral fragment and compress the fracture.

Caution

Check for rotational errors.
Closed advancing of the wire through the distal fragment of diaphyseal fractures is not always possible.

- Cut off, shorten, and bend the free wire ends (▶ Fig. 10.26f).
- Suture the periosteum and skin.

10.11.2 Antegrade Intramedullary Procedure for Proximal and Middle Phalanx Fractures

- Make ulnar and radial stab incisions in the skin over the radial/ulnar dorsum of the base of the proximal or middle phalanx (▶ Fig. 10.27a).
- Make a short longitudinal incision in the oblique or transverse part of the intertendinous part of the extensor aponeurosis.
- Expose the base of the bone by blunt dissection with a hemostat (▶ Fig. 10.27b).
- Open the medullary cavity with an awl or drill.
- Introduce the Kirschner wire or pin into the medullary cavity and advance it as far as the fracture (▶ Fig. 10.27c).
- Reduce the fracture under image intensifier control in both planes.
- Advance the Kirschner wire or pin until it is in distal metaphyseal subchondral position and compress the fracture (▶ Fig. 10.27d).
- Carry out the same procedure on the opposite side (▶ Fig. 10.27e).
- Take an intraoperative check X-ray and suture the skin.

10.11.3 Retrograde intramedullary Procedure for Proximal and Middle Phalanx Fractures

- Make dorsoradial and dorsoulnar stab incisions in the skin, distally over the proximal and middle phalanx but proximal to the distal or proximal interphalangeal joint.
- Make a longitudinal incision in the extensor tendon hood: radial and ulnar to the central slip; on the middle phalanx distally; and make parallel incisions radial and ulnar to the central slip on the proximal phalanx distally.

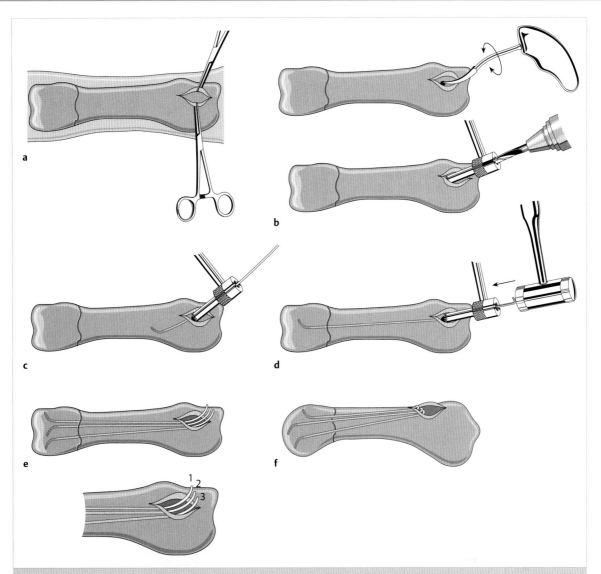

Fig. 10.26 Antegrade intramedullary pinning of metacarpal fractures. **(a)** Make a stab incision and expose the bone by blunt dissection. **(b)** Open the medullary cavity with an awl or drill. **(c)** Bend the distal blunt end of the pin slightly, introduce it into the medullary cavity. Push a long drill guide over the pin and bend the proximal end of the pin 90° in the direction of the bent distal end. **(d)** Under image intensifier control, hammer the intramedullary pin in as far as the fracture. The fracture is reduced, the pin is threaded into the distal fragment, bridging the fracture gap. The pin is positioned in the distal subcortical end of the bone. The fracture is compressed. **(e)** Repeat the procedure with the second and third pins. **(f)** After checking the position of the fracture, especially rotation, compress the fracture, shorten the distal ends, and bury the ends subcutaneously.

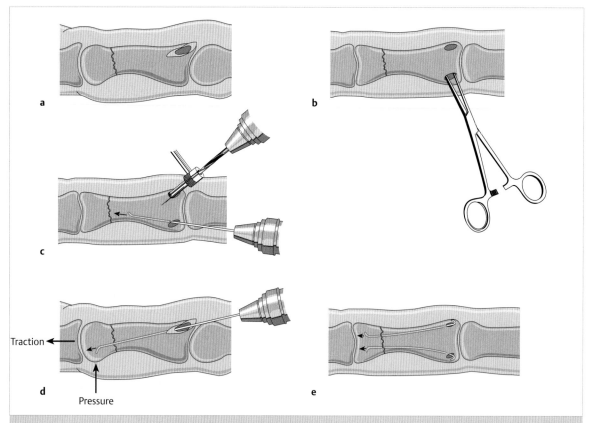

Fig. 10.27 Antegrade intramedullary pinning of proximal and middle phalanx fractures. **(a)** Dorsoradial and dorsoulnar stab skin incision, lateral view. **(b)** Expose the extensor tendon by blunt dissection and make a short longitudinal incision lateral to the central slip, to expose the base of the bone. View from above. **(c)** Open the medullary cavity with an awl or drill, introduce a slightly bent pin, blunt distally, and advance it as far as the fracture. **(d)** Reduce the fracture and advance the pin under image intensifier control in two planes until it attains a subchondral position in the distal fragment. Compress the fracture. **(e)** Repeat the procedure on the opposite side and bury the wires subcutaneously after shortening them.

⚠

Caution

Do not divide the lateral slip. Access to the proximal phalanx dorsally is at the level of the origin of the collateral ligaments and accessory collateral ligament. Preserve the joint capsule.

- Expose the bone by blunt dissection with a hemostat (► Fig. 10.28a).
- Open the medullary cavity with an awl or drill (► Fig. 10.28b).

- Introduce the Kirschner wire or pin into the medullary cavity under image intensifier control in both planes and advance it as far as the fracture gap (► Fig. 10.28c).
- Reduce the fracture under image intensifier control in both planes.
- Advance the intramedullary fixation material until it is in proximal metaphyseal subchondral position and compress the fracture (► Fig. 10.28d).
- Take an intraoperative check X-ray and suture the skin.

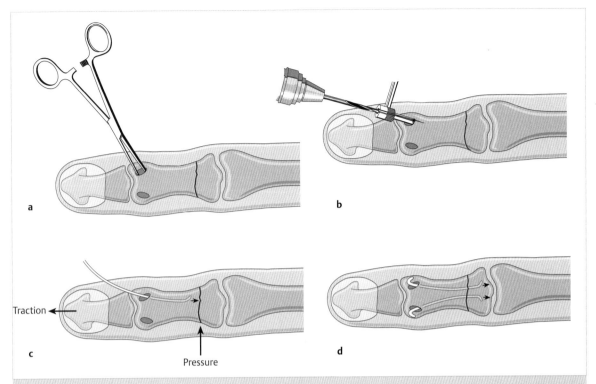

Fig. 10.28 Retrograde intramedullary pinning of proximal and middle phalanx fractures. **(a)** Make dorsoradial and dorsoulnar stab incisions distally over the proximal or middle phalanx; make a longitudinal incision in the extensor tendon outside the lateral slip. Expose the proximal subcapital part of the bone dorsal to the collateral ligaments and proximal to the joint capsule. **(b)** Open the medullary cavity with an awl or drill. **(c)** Advance a pin, bent slightly beforehand and blunt distally, as far as the fracture. **(d)** Reduce the fracture under image intensifier control and advance the pin in the medullary cavity as far as the metaphyseal region. Repeat this on the opposite side. After shortening the pins, bury the ends subcutaneously.

10.12 External Fixator

10.12.1 Indications, Advantages, and Disadvantages

If internal fixation is not indicated because of the type of injury, an external fixator usually offers the possibility of fixation with motion stability.

▶ **Indications.** The indications for an external fixator include:
- Open fractures
- Closed comminuted fractures
- Fracture-dislocations that can be reduced by ligamentotaxis
- Infections of bone, joint and/or soft tissue
- Complex soft tissue and/or bone defects
- Traumatic bone defects
- Fractures in which soft tissue damage can be expected
- Following tumor resection

The possibilities for using the different elements of an external fixator, including frame construction, offer great variability.

▶ **Advantages**
- Early motion stability with only minimal soft tissue trauma
- The fracture and fracture hematoma are left untouched
- Wound inspections and dressing changes are unproblematic
- A change of procedure is possible after the soft tissues have been treated
- No infection-promoting metallic foreign bodies are present in the fracture region.
- Early mobilization of uninvolved joints promotes wound healing and prevents decreased range of mobility
- Bone graft interposition into defects is possible

▶ **Disadvantages.** Infection and/or loosening of the pins Often, not accepted by patients

10.12.2 Construction Possibilities and Placement

▶ **Construct elements.** The individual elements of an external fixator are (▶ Fig. 10.29):

- Pin = Steinmann pin = Schanz screw = Kirschner wire (1 in ▶ Fig. 10.29).
- Holding pin clamp = connection clamp = articulation coupling (2 in ▶ Fig. 10.29)
- Guide, bridging, or connecting rods/tubes/bars (3 in ▶ Fig. 10.29).
- Universal joint for rod/tube-to-rod/tube coupling = articulation element (4 in ▶ Fig. 10.29)

▶ **Constructions.** The structural elements allow a variety of uses:

- Unilateral clamp fixator, single bone (▶ Fig. 10.30a, b)
- Joint-bridging in two bones (▶ Fig. 10.30c)
- Frame in one plane, single bone (▶ Fig. 10.30d)
- Frames in three planes, one or more bones, for example, V-shaped (▶ Fig. 10.30e), tent-shaped (▶ Fig. 10.30f)
- Joint-bridging in two bones (▶ Fig. 10.30g)
- Joint-bridging in multiple bones (▶ Fig. 10.30h)
- Double rod, multiple rod assemblage

In principle, threaded pins or Steinmann pins, Schanz screws, and Kirschner wires are inserted in the bone(s) and linked to each other by guide, bridging, or connecting rods, articulation elements, connecting clamps, and joints for coupling enable three-dimensional constructions.

▶ **Locations.** Pins and Steinmann pins, Schanz screws, and Kirschner wires are placed in the metacarpals and phalanges to protect nerves, vessels, tendons, and ligaments within certain areas (▶ Fig. 10.31a, b).

10.12.3 Procedure

- Make a stab skin incision.
- Dissect bluntly down to the periosteum.
- Make a stab incision in the periosteum.
- Place the drill or guide sleeve on the periosteum.
- Predrill if necessary.

Note

The size of the drill depends on the construct elements, namely:
- ○ Pin = Steinmann pin → drill diameter
- ○ Schanz screw → thread core diameter

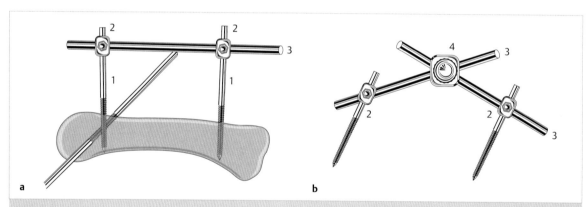

Fig. 10.29 External fixator elements. The individual elements of an external fixator are given different names, depending on the manufacturer, though they have the same function.
1: Pin = Steinmann pin = Schanz screw = Kirschner wire; these elements are usually inserted after predrilling or are drilled in directly.
2: Holding pin clamp = connection clamp = articulation coupling; their function is to connect the elements labeled 1 with the rods/tubes/bars labeled 3.
3: Guide, bridging, or connecting rods/tubes/ bars.
4: Universal joint for rod/tube-to-rod/tube coupling = articulation element; their function is to allow variable fixed connection of the rods labeled 3 at any angle.

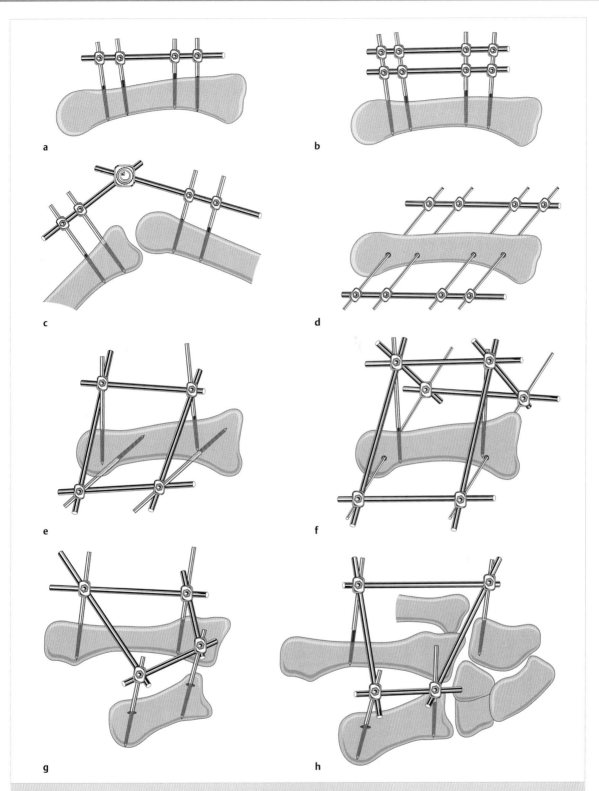

Fig. 10.30 External fixator constructions. Very varied constructions are possible using combinations of the listed elements. These are adapted to special situations. **(a)** Unilateral in one bone. **(b)** Unilateral in one bone with double rod. **(c)** Unilateral joint-bridging in two bones. **(d)** Single bone frame construction. **(e)** V-frame in one bone. **(f)** Tent frame in one bone. **(g)** Frame construction in two bones. **(h)** Frame construction in multiple bones.

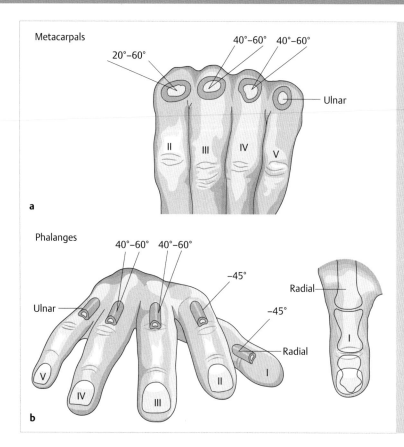

Metacarpals

40°–60° 40°–60°

20°–60°

Ulnar

II   III   IV   V

a

Phalanges

40°–60° 40°–60°

–45°

Radial

Ulnar

–45°

Radial

V   IV   III   II   I

I

b

Fig. 10.31 To protect soft tissues and structures, especially extensor tendons, the elements required for the external fixator are applied only in certain regions. These differ according to the individual rays.
(a) Suitable sites in the metacarpal region.
(b) Suitable sites in the phalanges.

- Introduce the pin into the fragment (▶ Fig. 10.32a)
- Cross the center of the medullary space as perpendicularly to the bone surface as possible.
- Grip both cortices, but for unilateral assemblage place the tip just in the opposite cortex and do not allow it to project into the soft tissues.
- For frames: Carefully penetrate the contralateral soft tissues bluntly until the tip is palpable beneath the skin. Then make a stab incision in the skin and advance the pin further (▶ Fig. 10.32b).
- Insert the second pin in the opposite fragment and make sure that the pins are aligned in one plane (▶ Fig. 10.32c).
- Mount a connecting rod on the two pins by means of a holding pin clamp.
- After preparation of the uni- or bicortical frame, reduce the fracture under image intensifier control in all planes. Correct rotation is important.
- Following reduction, tighten the holding pin clamps on the connecting rod for provisional fixation.
- For a two-dimensional or three-dimensional assemblage, thread the necessary number of connecting pin clamps onto the connecting rod beforehand.
- If additional pins are placed in the fragments, use a drill guide or double drill guide (▶ Fig. 10.32d).

Practical Tip

It is difficult to place four pins parallel to one another for a connecting rod. It is better to use one connecting rod per fragment and, following reduction, to fix the two connecting rods by articulation elements (▶ Fig. 10.32e). Intraoperative radiographic imaging is easier using carbon fiber rods.

- Shorten the projecting pins.
- Reduce the size of the skin incision by suture.
- Apply a dressing.

In the case of extra-articular fractures close to joints, intra-articular fractures, and avulsion fractures, adequate fracture reduction can often be achieved by ligamentotaxis. In this situation, however, external fixation by means of a splint only is often insufficient. Stable fixation of the reduction can often be ensured by a *multi-bone frame assemblage*. Examples include Bennett fractures, Rolando fractures of the thumb, and wrist fractures.

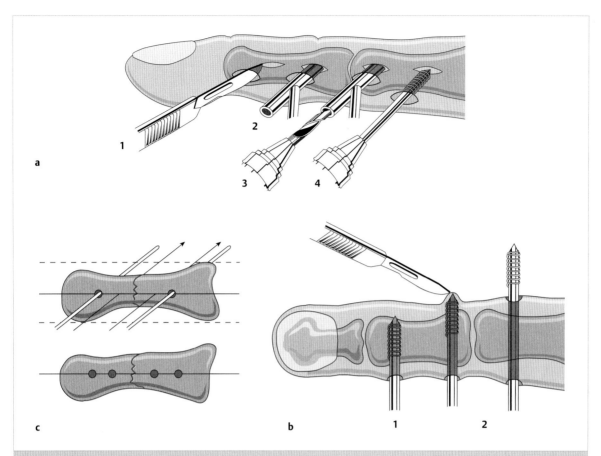

Fig. 10.32 Application of an external fixator. **(a)** When constructing intraosseous elements, the same procedure is usually followed. 1: Stab skin incision and blunt exposure of the bone; 2: application of a drill sleeve; 3: drilling of a hole of correct size, if necessary; 4: introduction of a pin or Steinmann pin, Schanz screw, or Kirschner wire. **(b)** For unilateral constructions, the intraosseous element should just touch the opposite cortex without perforating it (1). For a frame construction, both cortices are first drilled through and the stabilizing element is passed through the bone until it nearly perforates the skin. This can be brought out fully through a stab incision (2). **(c)** For a frame construction it is advisable to place two intraosseous elements per fragment. It is difficult to place these four elements in the same plane and achieve normal rotation.

Continued ▶

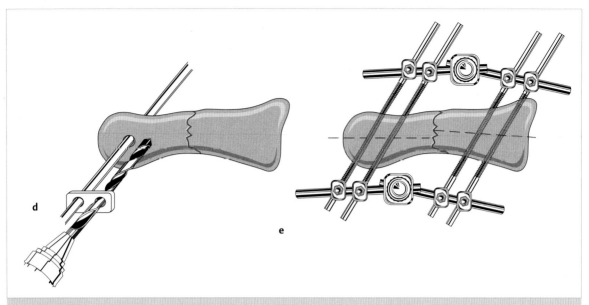

Fig. 10.32 *(Continued)* **(d)** Use of a drill guide or double drill guide within a fragment makes it easier to place the second element in the correct axis. **(e)** The following procedure greatly facilitates construction of a frame: Two intraosseous elements per fragment are first constructed and then connecting rods/tubes are applied on both sides to join the intraosseous elements. After reducing the fracture and checking the axis and rotation, these are fixed with universal joint for rod/tube-to-rod/tube coupling or articulation elements.

10.13 Adaptive Fixation

10.13.1 Overview

It is not possible to achieve sufficient early motion stability for all fractures in the hand by internal fixation. In such cases, nonoperative management should be considered first. However, if this appears inadvisable, adaptive fixation is an option.

The possible operation methods are:
- Percutaneous Kirschner wire fixation
- Ender–Hintringer hooked wire
- Ender–Hintringer plug method
- Retrograde single-wire technique
- Ishiguro operation (extension block pinning)
- Percutaneous transfixation

The soft tissue layer in the hand is very thin. Particularly in the fingers, the functional structures—that is, nerves, vessels, tendons, sliding tissue, and ligaments—are very close to each other. Protection of these structures is a priority.

If other operative techniques are not possible, adaptive fixation by means of *Kirschner wire fixation* is the least invasive option with the least trauma for soft tissues. It is mainly used in the distal phalanx and metaphysis of the phalanges. With smaller avulsion fractures, it is sometimes not possible to achieve closed reduction prior to adaptive fixation. In these cases, open reduction is performed, followed by adaptive fixation if motion stability cannot be achieved.

Transfixation of two or more bones is an extended alternative method of treating fractures.

10.13.2 Percutaneous Kirschner Wire Fixation

Percutaneous Kirschner wire fixation can be regarded as a minimally invasive method. Because of the complicated anatomy, it is used mainly in the distal phalanx and in the metaphyseal region of the middle and proximal phalanges. It always requires additional external immobilization. The operation must be performed under X-ray control.

- As far as possible, always drill from the smaller to the bigger fragment (▶ Fig. 10.33a).
- Two Kirschner wires should preferably be inserted:
  - Axial: two parallel wires (▶ Fig. 10.33b)
  - Crossed: the wires should cross outside the fracture gap (▶ Fig. 10.33c)
- In the distal phalanx, insert axial Kirschner wires from distal to proximal: drill under visual control following a fish mouth incision and exposure of the head of the phalanx (▶ Fig. 10.33d).
- Use the lowest possible drill speed to minimize heating.
- Whenever possible, avoid temporary joint transfixation by transarticular Kirschner wires because of the risk of thermal damage to cartilage.

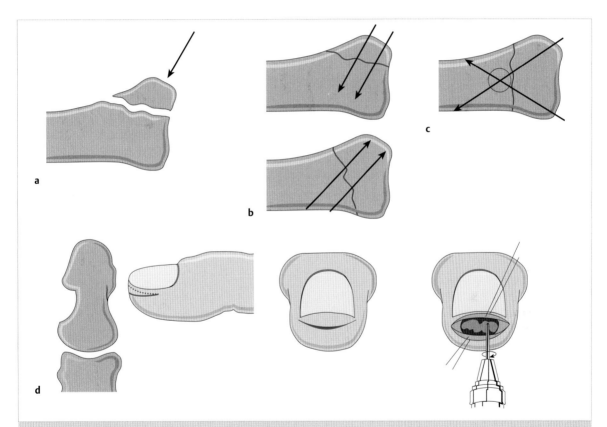

Fig. 10.33 Percutaneous Kirschner wire fixation. **(a)** When inserting percutaneous Kirschner wires, drilling must proceed from the smaller to the larger fragment as otherwise the wire will dislocate the smaller fragment during drilling. **(b)** To achieve more secure rotational stability, it is advisable to place two Kirschner wires parallel to one another, especially when the wires are in axial position. **(c)** If the wires are crossed, again on account of rotational stability, they should cross outside the fracture gap. **(d)** When drilling Kirschner wires into the distal phalanx from distal to proximal, the distal phalanx should first be exposed by a fish-mouth incision so that the wires can be placed under visual control. Experience has shown that Kirschner wires inserted blind have a tendency to slide off the hard cortex of the distal end of the phalanx in palmar direction.

Continued ▶

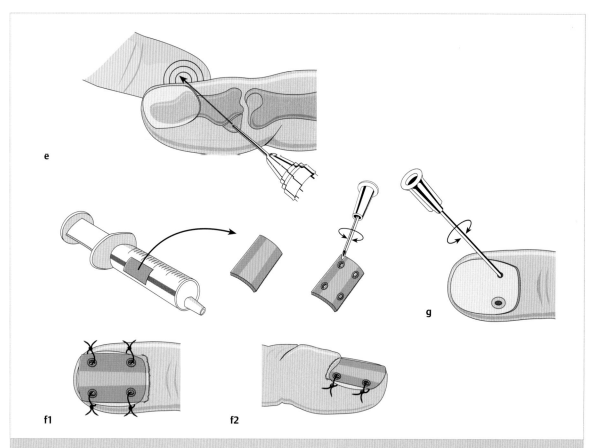

Fig. 10.33 (*Continued*) **(e)** For spatial orientation, it is helpful for the surgeon to aim toward a free fingertip on the opposite side and to drill under image intensification. This avoids unnecessary repeated drilling. **(f)** The nail plate has a good supporting function in distal phalanx fractures and must therefore be replaced by an artificial nail when the fracture involves loss of the nail plate. A good substitute can be provided by an "artificial nail plate" cut from a sterile syringe. Holes can be made in it with a size no. 1 needle so that the artificial nail can be fixed with sutures. These holes also allow drainage of any subungual hematomas. **(g)** When the nail plate is preserved but there is a subungual hematoma, perforation of the nail plate can be achieved readily without anesthetic by making trephine holes with a size no. 1 needle. Better drainage is obtained than with the traditional method using a heated paper clip, as there is no heat coagulation.

- The nail plate has an important support function in peripheral and diaphyseal fractures of the distal phalanx. If the nail plate is lost, temporary splinting by an artificial nail is required (▶ Fig. 10.33f).
- Subungual hematomas must be trephined. Pierce the nail plate with a sterile size no. 1 needle; it is possible without anesthetic (▶ Fig. 10.33g).
- Nail bed injuries must be sutured with the finest absorbable sutures.

10.13.3 Procedure for Ender–Hintringer Hooked Wire

- The avulsed side of the phalangeal base is reduced percutaneously with a needle and the fracture is fixed by pressure on the needle (▶ Fig. 10.34a).
- Advance the Kirschner wire through the fragment via the needle (▶ Fig. 10.344b).
- Drill through the fracture and cortex beyond the fracture until the Kirschner wire perforates the soft tissues (▶ Fig. 10.34c).

- Continue to drill the Kirschner wire, grasp it, remove the needle, and bend the end of the wire into a hook shape on the side of the fracture. Make a stab incision (▶ Fig. 10.34d).
- Under traction, grip the fragment with the hook, and reduce and fix it (▶ Fig. 10.34e).
- Bend the other end over a dressing or plastic disc under traction and secure it with a compressed lead shot (▶ Fig. 10.34e).

10.13.4 Procedure for Ender–Hintringer Plug Method

- Make a stab incision on the extensor side near the central slip of the tendon at the level of the middle phalanx shaft (▶ Fig. 10.35a).
- Drill a hole at least 2 mm in diameter obliquely and tangentially from distal to proximal as far as the medullary cavity (▶ Fig. 10.35b).

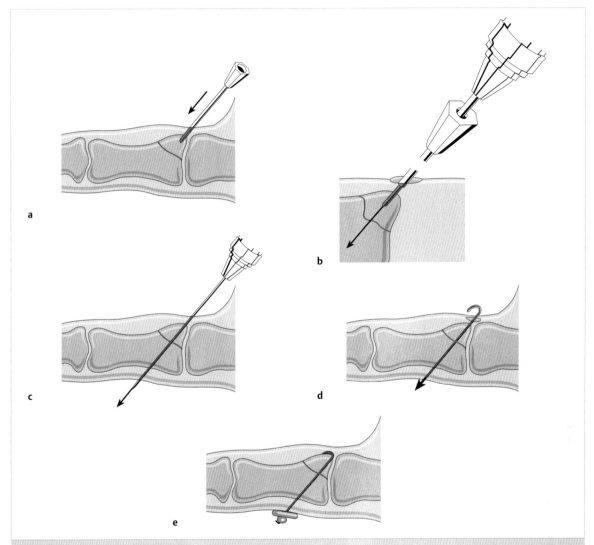

Fig. 10.34 Ender–Hintringer hooked wire. **(a)** The avulsed fragment is reduced by pushing it with a percutaneously introduced cannula of large diameter. **(b)** The fragment is fixed with a Kirschner wire through the cannula. **(c)** The wire is drilled through the cortex and soft tissues beyond the fracture and out through the skin. **(d)** After withdrawing the cannula that is acting as a drill guide, the wire is bent into a hook shape at the end from which it was inserted. A stab skin incision is made at the wire's entry site. **(e)** The wire is pulled through the incision from the other end using rotating movements until the hook has gripped the fragment. Using traction, the wire is fixed and secured on the exit side over a dressing and plastic disk with a compressed lead shot.

- Bend the blunt end of a Kirschner wire, 1 mm in diameter, into a hook.
- After threading the hook into the medullary cavity, push the depressed basal fragments in proximal direction (▶ Fig. 10.35c).
- Rotate the bent end in a circle so that the entire basal surface is pushed proximally; use the trochlea of the adjacent articular plane to form a stepless articular base by pushing the comminuted fragments against the trochlea (▶ Fig. 10.35d)
- If the fragments shift laterally, reduce these with ligamentotaxis by longitudinal traction on the finger.
- Insert Kirschner wires percutaneously in a starlike pattern from all four sides—ulnar, radial, oblique palmar (note the neurovascular bundle), and oblique dorsal—to support the aligned fragments (▶ Fig. 10.35e).
- Pass the wire through the bigger palmar shear fragment obliquely from the palmar side, press it against the aligned basal fragments, and then drill through it until the Kirschner wire perforates the soft tissues of the opposite side (▶ Fig. 10.35f).
- Change the drill to the other end and drill the Kirschner wire from the extensor side until the end of the wire grips the palmar cortex of the sheared-off fragment (▶ Fig. 10.35g).
- Move the Kirschner wire to subcutaneous position on the extensor side (▶ Fig. 10.35h).
- Immobilize in a splint for 4 to 6 weeks.

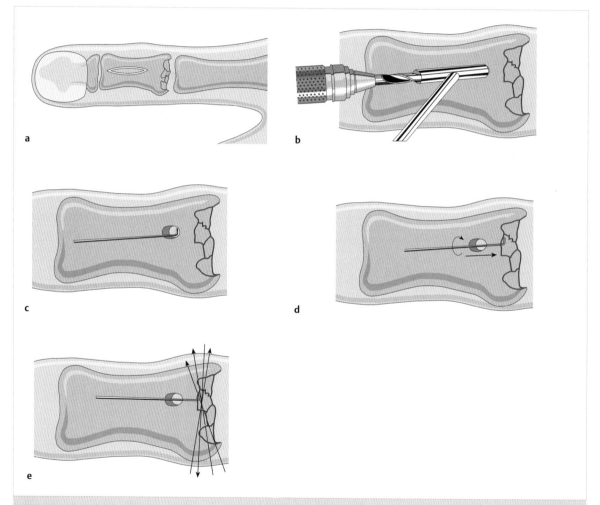

Fig. 10.35 Ender–Hintringer plug method. **(a)** A stab skin incision is made in the middle third of the extensor side and a short longitudinal incision is made parallel and lateral to the central slip, to obtain access to the shaft. **(b)** The medullary cavity is entered by drilling tangentially an oblique hole at least 2 mm in diameter, from distal to proximal. **(c)** The end of a 1-mm Kirschner wire is bent in such a way that the hook can be introduced into the medullary cavity through the 2 mm hole. The fracture fragments at the base are pushed proximally with the blunt end. **(d)** The wire is rotated in a circle within the medullary cavity and the fragments are pushed against the articular head until the basal joint surface is restored without a step-off. **(e)** If the fragments move laterally, they are reduced by ligamentotaxis using longitudinal traction. After the joint surface has been reconstituted, Kirschner wires are placed percutaneously parallel to the joint surface in a starlike pattern so that they prevent the fragments from moving back distally.

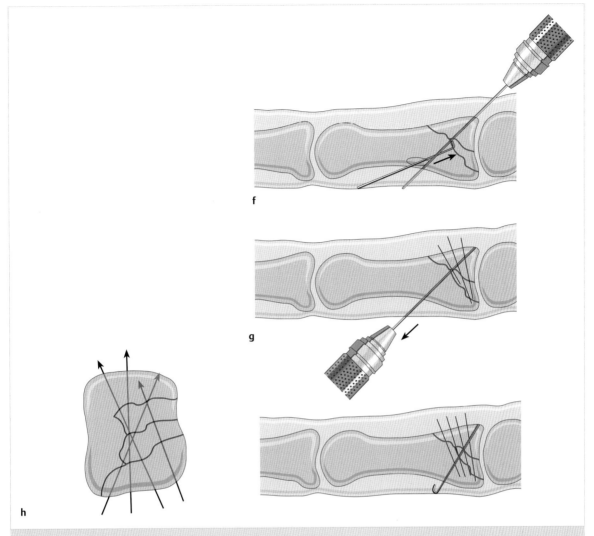

Fig. 10.35 *(Continued)* **(f)** Larger edge fragments are supported in the medullary cavity and drilled percutaneously with a Kirschner wire. The wire is advanced until it perforates the soft tissues and skin on the opposite side. **(g)** After moving the drill to the other end of the wire that has perforated the skin, the wire is drilled through distally until the proximal end of the wire just makes contact with the cortex of the edge fragment. **(h)** After bending the end of the stabilizing wire, the end is buried subcutaneously.

10.13.5 Retrograde Single-Wire Technique

- With the distal interphalangeal joint in maximum flexion, drill a double-pointed Kirschner wire percutaneously across the fracture in the medullary cavity parallel to the dorsal cortex of the distal phalanx to beyond the fingertip (▶ Fig. 10.36a).
- Switch the drill position and drill in proximal direction until the proximal tip of the Kirschner wire lies just in the fracture.

- Reduce the fracture under image intensifier control with the distal interphalangeal joint in maximum extension and external pressure on the dorsal avulsed fracture of the phalangeal base.
- After reduction of the fracture, drill the wire back in proximal direction through the dorsal fragment and distal interphalangeal joint to transfix the joint in hyperextension while fixing the fracture (▶ Fig. 10.36b).
- Move the Kirschner wire to a subcutaneous position in the fingertip.

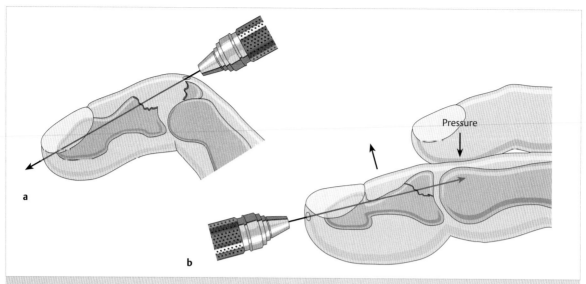

a

b

Pressure

Fig. 10.36 Retrograde single-wire technique. **(a)** Dorsal fragments resulting from bony extensor tendon avulsion fractures are usually exposed. The distal interphalangeal joint is flexed maximally and a double-pointed Kirschner wire is drilled percutaneously from proximal and dorsal through the fracture into the medullary space of the distal phalanx parallel to the dorsal cortex until the tip of the wire perforates the fingertip. **(b)** The drill is switched to the distal end of the wire. The wire is drawn distally until the proximal tip is distal to the fracture gap. With the distal interphalangeal joint in maximum extension, the fracture is reduced by simultaneous dorsal pressure. The intramedullary Kirschner wire is now drilled proximally so that it passes through the fracture fragment, at the same time transfixing the joint in extension. The axial wire is moved to subcutaneous position in the fingertip.

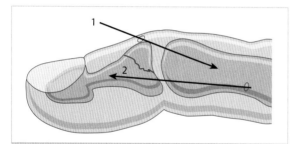

Fig. 10.37 Ishiguro operation, extension block pinning. Following maximum flexion of the distal interphalangeal joint, the dorsal avulsed fragment is drawn as far distally as possible via the reserve extensor apparatus. An intra-articular Kirschner wire is drilled percutaneously as far distally as possible for passive retention of the fragment (1). The joint is then transfixed temporarily with an oblique Kirschner wire (2) with the distal interphalangeal joint in maximum extension for optimal reduction of the fracture. A minor extension deficit can be tolerated.

10.13.6 Ishiguro Operation / Extension Block Pinning

- Reduce the bony fragment at the dorsal base of the distal phalanx by maximum flexion of the distal interphalangeal joint.

- Insert a Kirschner wire percutaneously into the head of the middle phalanx from distal dorsal to proximal palmar, blocking the avulsed fragment and blocking the action of the extensor tendon (1 in ► Fig. 10.37).
- This is followed by maximum extension of the distal phalanx, thus reducing the fragment into the fracture bed.
- Fix the distal phalanx in extension by oblique percutanous joint transfixation by means of a second Kirschner wire (2 in ► Fig. 10.37); minimal flexion can be tolerated.

10.13.7 Transfixation with Kirschner Wires

When avulsion fractures become subluxed or dislocated by tendon traction—usually at the base of the first and fifth metacarpals—the tendon traction can be neutralized by percutaneous transfixation.
- After reduction of the fracture under traction by ligamentotaxis, drill a Kirschner wire percutaneously through the proximal shaft toward neighboring bones.
- Drill completely through the cortices of both bones.

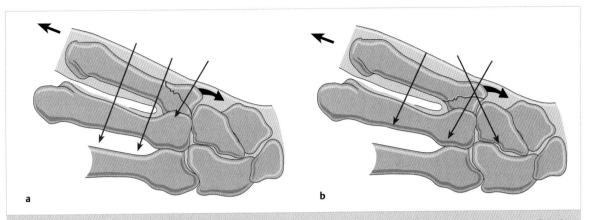

Fig. 10.38 Transfixation with Kirschner wires. **(a)** Using longitudinal traction, the fracture that has been dislocated because of tendon traction is reduced and held in reduced position by Kirschner wires placed through the neighboring bones. **(b)** Variations in all directions are possible.

Practical Tip

It is necessary to aim precisely at the neighboring bone, as the direction can no longer be corrected after drilling through the second cortex of the bone.

- Always insert two Kirschner wires for secure stabilization of the bones. The further distally that the second wire is placed, the more stable the transfixation, but this is a difficult technique.

- When the second Kirschner wire meets the opposite bone, this is readily palpable and confirms that the direction is correct (▶ Fig. 10.38a, b).
- The Kirschner wires are usually buried subcutaneously after shortening. They can only be left above skin level if the wound is monitored regularly.
- The wires should be removed as soon as possible.

10.14 Temporary Percutaneous Joint Transfixation

10.14.1 Procedure

- Drill the Kirschner wire, if possible in an oblique diagonal direction (▶ Fig. 10.39a, b).
- If axial, introduce two parallel Kirschner wires to achieve rotational stability (see Chapter 10.13.2 "Percutaneous Kirschner Wire Fixation").
- Drill at the lowest possible speed to avoid thermal damage to cartilage.

Note

Transfixation of joints is also possible in the carpal bones, with all variations.

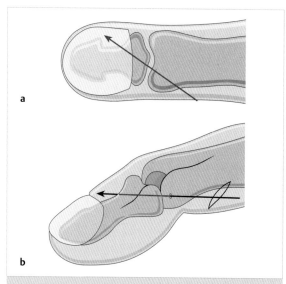

Fig. 10.39 Percutaneous temporary joint transfixation. Under image intensifier control, a Kirschner wire is drilled obliquely through the joint percutaneously using a low drill speed to avoid thermal injury. **(a)** View from above. **(b)** Dorsolateral view.

10.15 Dynamic Distraction External Fixation

Fractures at the base of the middle phalanx following axial compression often result in subluxation and dislocation of the middle phalanx from the proximal phalanx due to the proximal longitudinal traction of the tendons. In addition, the base of the middle phalanx is quite often either depressed or destroyed by a comminuted fracture so that internal fixation is not possible. These situations can be managed effectively by dynamic distraction external fixation. This dynamic treatment allows immediate postoperative active physical therapy to prevent decreased range of motion, especially in the proximal interphalangeal joint. Early exercise also allows good remodeling of the proximal joint surface of the middle phalanx.

10.15.1 Suzuki Operation / Dynamic Distraction External Fixation

- Start by drilling a long Kirschner wire (W1) percutaneously through the head of the proximal phalanx from ulnar to radial in the rotational center of the joint (▶ Fig. 10.40a).
- Drill a second Kirschner wire (W2) percutanously through the center of rotation of the middle phalanx from ulnar to radial.
- Drill a third Kirschner wire (W3) through the midshaft of the middle phalanx.
- All three Kirschner wires are parallel to one another and perpendicular to the axis of the finger (▶ Fig. 10.40b).
- Bend both ends of the first wire (W1) distally along the axis of the finger, palmar to the third wire (W3) and palmar to the midshaft Kirschner wire (W3).
- At the level of the fingertip bend the first wire (W1) into a hook on both sides to accept a rubber band.
- After shortening the most distal Kirschner wire (W2) on the radial and ulnar sides, bend it into a hook to accept a rubber band.
- The midshaft wire (W3) is placed dorsal to the wire (W1), shortened and the ends are bent in a palmar direction. This Kirschner wire (W3) serves as fulcrum to support the long frame of the first wire (W1).
- A rubber band is attached between the hooks on either side so that the middle phalanx is under traction relative to the proximal phalanx (▶ Fig. 10.40c, d).
- Flexion and extension in the proximal interphalangeal joint are possible by rotating the wire in the head of the proximal phalanx
- To avoid skin infections due to the rotating wire, a small tube can also be placed in the head of the proximal phalanx over the wire (W1) so that it rotates in the tube, thereby protecting the skin (▶ Fig. 10.40e).

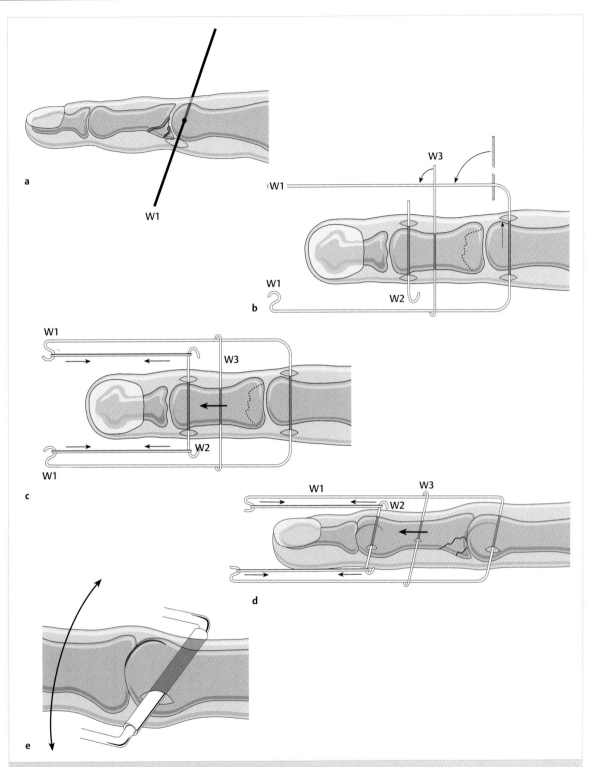

Fig. 10.40 Dynamic distraction external fixation according to Suzuki. **(a)** A first Kirschner wire (W1) is drilled transversely through the head of the proximal phalanx in the rotational center of the joint **(b)** A second Kirschner wire (W2) is placed through the rotational center of the head of the middle phalanx, whereas the third wire (W3) is drilled through the midshaft of the middle phalanx. All three wires are parallel to one another, perpendicular to the axis of the phalanx. After bending both sides of the first wire (W1) parallel to the long axis of the finger, this wire (W1) is shortened outside the fingertip; the ends are bent into a hook. The ends of the most distal Kirschner wire (W2) are also formed into hooks after shortening; both to accept a rubber band later. The Kirschner wire (W3) in the midshaft is shortened, bent dorsally and located palmar to the first Kirschner wire (W1) to act as a fulcrum to support the long frame of the first wire (W1). **(c)** The hooks are placed under tension bilaterally using rubber bands so that the middle phalanx is drawn distally relative to the proximal phalanx (view from above). **(d)** Lateral view of the distraction. **(e)** To protect the soft tissues, especially the skin near the head of the proximal phalanx, which is at risk of infection due to rotation of the Kirschner wire, a small tube can be passed over the first transosseous wire and advanced through the head of the proximal phalanx.

The commercially available dynamic intradigital mini external fixator is based on the same biomechanical principle.

10.16 Pull-out Barbed Wire Suture / Lengemann Suture

Dislocated bone and ligament avulsion fractures with fragments that do not allow stable fixation can usually be reduced and fixed with a removable Lengemann suture. There is no compression of the fracture. The bony fragments are simply approximated. Excessive pressure on the soft tissues by fixation on the opposite side of the fracture bears the risk of pressure necrosis and infection. Supporting it by a small tube on the periosteum may be helpful (see ▶ Fig. 10.41h).

This method has generally become out of fashion and should only be used in isolated cases. It is most commonly used for dislocated bone and ligament avulsions involving the ulnar collateral ligament at the base of the proximal phalanx of the thumb (gamekeeper's thumb).

10.16.1 Procedure

- Under Under visual control or percutaneously, drill through the avulsed fragment and fracture surface toward the opposite cortex using a low drill speed; then drill through the opposite cortex and soft tissues (▶ Fig. 10.41a).
- Place a cannula on the tip of the Kirschner wire and push the cannula through the shaft, fracture, and avulsed fragment by withdrawing the Kirschner wire while pressing on the cannula (▶ Fig. 10.41b).
- Introduce the tip of the Lengemann suture needle into the cannula and draw it through the bone to the other side of the finger by withdrawing the cannula (▶ Fig. 10.41c, d).
- Make a stab incision, dissect the avulsed fragment, reduce it and place the barb of the Lengemann suture on the fragment (▶ Fig. 10.41e).

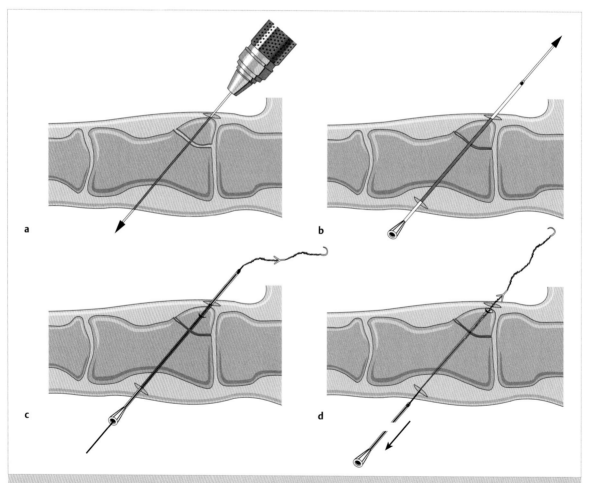

Fig. 10.41 Pull-out barbed wire suture according to Lengemann. **(a)** Drill percutaneously through the avulsed edge fragment, at the same time reducing it by pressure if the size of the fragment allows this. The Kirschner wire is drilled through the cortex opposite to the fracture and through the skin. **(b)** A cannula is placed over the drilled Kirschner wire and pushed through the bone over the Kirschner wire. **(c)** The straight needle of the Lengemann suture is now passed through the bone using the cannula. **(d)** As the cannula is withdrawn, the needle is drawn through the bone to the opposite side. Make a stab incision at the suture entry site and expose the edge fragment.

- Under traction, fix the fragment in the fracture site and maintain the approximation by pulling the wire to the opposite side (▶ Fig. 10.41e).
- When the avulsed fragments are too small to drill owing to the risk of fracturing them, place the barb directly at the insertion of the ligament (▶ Fig. 10.41f).
- Maintain the traction by a compressed lead shot over a dressing and plastic disk. Use a washer to protect the soft tissues (▶ Fig. 10.41g).

- To avoid pressure complications of the soft tissues, pass a small tube over the Lengemann suture; after making a stab incision place it on the cortex and maintain traction by means of a lead shot (▶ Fig. 10.41h).
- Bury the proximal wire subcutaneously.
- Remove the Lengemann suture after the fracture has healed. The distal lead shot is removed and, under anesthetic nerve block, the transosseous wire and barb are removed by traction on the proximal end of the wire.

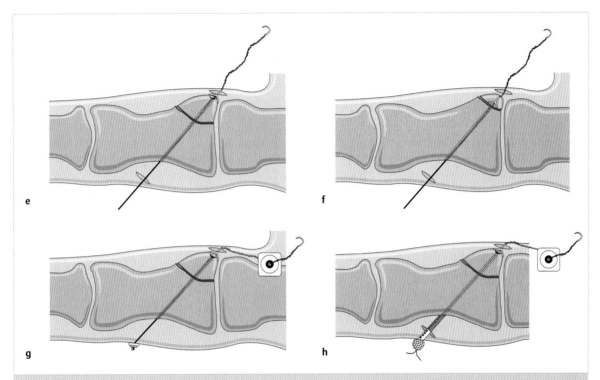

Fig. 10.41 *(Continued)* **(e)** The barb is positioned on the cortex. Reduce the avulsed edge fragment with traction using the barb and fix the fracture. **(f)** When the fragment is small, just pass the barb through the soft tissues, as close as possible to the bony fragment. **(g)** The reduction and suture traction are maintained by a compressed lead shot over a dressing and plastic washer. The proximal wire suture is drawn subcutaneously in proximal direction and through the skin, where it is likewise fixed over a dressing. **(h)** To avoid soft tissue damage due to pressure of the plastic disk on the skin, it is useful to pass the Lengemann suture through a tube. The tube used for support is advanced through a stab incision over the suture as far as the periosteum. This avoids pressure on the skin and soft tissues and the risk of complications is lower.

10.17 Hook Plate / Pronged Plate

10.17.1 Procedure

- Make a **Y**-shaped skin incision over the dorsum of the distal interphalangeal joint (► Fig. 10.42a).
- Expose the dorsal fracture of the base of the distal phalanx with the attached extensor tendon (► Fig. 10.42b).
- Reduce the fracture anatomically. If necessary fix the fragment temporarily with a fine Kirschner wire. Be aware of the risk of fracturing the fragment.

- Apply the plate with the hook holding the proximal fragment, then fix the plate with an appropriate screw; place the screw parallel to the joint surface (dorsal to palmar) (► Fig. 10.42c, d).
- If necessary, elevate the nail bed from the bone and push the plate under it.

Caution

It is essential to avoid damaging the proximal nail matrix as otherwise the nail plate will become deformed. **Place the plate beneath the nail matrix.**

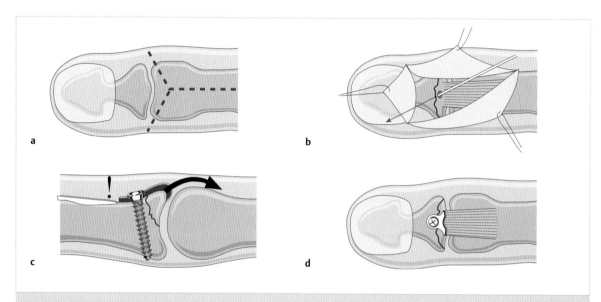

Fig. 10.42 Hook plate. **(a)** Y-shaped access to the dorsal distal interphalangeal joint. **(b)** Exposure of the dorsal basal fracture and reduction; temporary fixation by a fine Kirschner wire. **(c)** The plate is applied and fixed with a screw. The Kirschner wire is removed; lateral view. The nail matrix must never be compressed as this leads to nail plate deformities. If necessary, elevate the nail bed from the bone and push the plate under it. **(d)** Plate and screw fixation seen from above.

10.18 Absorbable pins

Internal fixation of intra-articular osteochondral fractures is often not possible with screws, either because the head of the screw would protrude into the load-bearing area of the joint surface or because of the risk of fragmentation of the osteochondral chip. Such fractures can be approximated by absorbable polymer pins, occasionally combined with fibrin glue.

As this is a purely adaptive fixation, external immobilization is required postoperatively. Full restoration of function may not be expected.

10.18.1 Procedure

- Open the joint (▶ Fig. 10.43a).
- Reduce the osteochondral fracture, possibly using fibrin glue.
- If possible, drill at least two diverging holes through the fragment and fragment bed of sufficient length and matching the pin diameter (▶ Fig. 10.43b).
- Insert the absorbable pins into the drill holes (▶ Fig. 10.43c).
- Shorten the pins at the level of the joint surface (▶ Fig. 10.43c)

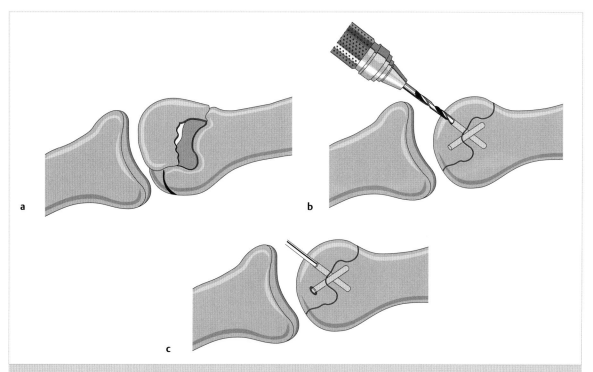

Fig. 10.43 Internal fixation with absorbable pins. **(a)** Extensive, intra-articular dislocated distal osteochondral fracture. **(b)** Appearance after reduction, with diverging holes drilled through the ostechondral fragment and fragment bed. **(c)** The pins are inserted into the holes and shortened at the level of the joint surface.

Chapter 11

Further Reading

11 Further Reading

11.1 Chapter 1: Introduction

Anakwe RE, Aitken SA, Cowie JG, Middleton SD, Court-Brown CM. The epidemiology of fractures of the hand and the influence of social deprivation. J Hand Surg Eur Vol 2011; 36: 62–65

Bartelmann U, Kotas J, Landsleitner B. Causes for reoperations after osteosyntheses of finger and mid-hand fractures.[Article in German.] Handchir Mikrochir Plast Chir 1997; 29: 204–208

Chew EM, Chong AK. Hand fractures in children: epidemiology and misdiagnosis in a tertiary referral hospital. J Hand Surg Am 2012; 37: 1684–1688

Chung KC, Spilson SV. The frequency and epidemiology of hand and forearm fractures in the United States. J Hand Surg Am 2001; 26: 908–915

Emmett JE, Breck LW. A review and analysis of 11,000 fractures seen in a private practice of orthopaedic surgery, 1937–1956. J Bone Joint Surg Am 1958; 40-A: 1169–1175

Feehan LM, Sheps SB. Incidence and demographics of hand fractures in British Columbia, Canada: a population-based study. J Hand Surg Am 2006; 31: 1068–1074

Frangen T, Muhr G, Kälicke T. Handwurzelfrakturen. Trauma Berufskrankh 2007; 9: 216–219

Leixnering M. Versorgung von Problemfrakturen an Finger und Mittelhand. JATROS Unfallchirurgie und Sporttraumatologie 2009; 4: 8–10

Meisinger C, Wildner M, Stieber J, Heier M, Sangha O, Döring A. Epidemiology of limb fractures.[Article in German.] Orthopäde 2002; 31: 92–99

Pun WK, Chow SP, So YC et al. A prospective study on 284 digital fractures of the hand. J Hand Surg Am 1989; 14: 474–481

Stanton JS, Dias JJ, Burke FD. Fractures of the tubular bones of the hand. J Hand Surg Eur Vol 2007; 32: 626–636

van Onselen EBH, Karim RB, Hage JJ, Ritt MJ. Prevalence and distribution of hand fractures. J Hand Surg [Br] 2003; 28: 491–495

Van Tassel DC, Owens BD, Wolf JM. Incidence estimates and demographics of scaphoid fracture in the U.S. population. J Hand Surg Am 2010; 35: 1242–1245

Yan YM, Zhang WP, Liao Y et al. [Analysis and prevention of the complications after treatment of metacarpal and phalangeal fractures with internal fixation] Zhongguo Gu Shang 2011; 24: 199–201(Abstract)

Young K, Greenwood A, MacQuillan A, Lee S, Wilson S. Paediatric hand fractures. J Hand Surg Eur Vol 2013; 38: 898–902

Zühlke A, Dietrich FE. Osteosynthesen am Handskelett. Handchir Mikrochir Plast Chir 2003; 35: A1–A45

11.2 Chapter 2: Biology of Fracture Healing

Augat P, Merk J, Wolf S, Claes L. Mechanical stimulation by external application of cyclic tensile strains does not effectively enhance bone healing. J Orthop Trauma 2001; 15: 54–60

Bishop NE, van Rhijn M, Tami I, Corveleijn R, Schneider E, Ito K. Shear does not necessarily inhibit bone healing. Clin Orthop Relat Res 2006; 443: 307–314

Dimitriou R, Jones E, McGonagle D, Giannoudis PV. Bone regeneration: current concepts and future directions. BMC Med 2011; 9: 66–73

Epari DR, Kassi J-P, Schell H, Duda GN. Timely fracture-healing requires optimization of axial fixation stability. J Bone Joint Surg Am 2007; 89: 1575–1585

Epari DR, Taylor WR, Heller MO, Duda GN. Mechanical conditions in the initial phase of bone healing. Clin Biomech (Bristol, Avon) 2006; 21: 646–655

Huang C, Ogawa R. Mechanotransduction in bone repair and regeneration. FASEB J 2010; 24: 3625–3632

Ilizarov GA. The tension-stress effect on the genesis and growth of tissues. Part I. The influence of stability of fixation and soft-tissue preservation. Clin Orthop Relat Res 1989: 249–281

Ingber DE. Tensegrity-based mechanosensing from macro to micro. Prog Biophys Mol Biol 2008; 97: 163–179

Ingber DE. Cellular mechanotransduction: putting all the pieces together again. FASEB J 2006; 20: 811–827

Isaksson H, Wilson W, van Donkelaar CC, Huiskes R, Ito K. Comparison of biophysical stimuli for mechano-regulation of tissue differentiation during fracture healing. J Biomech 2006; 39: 1507–1516

Ito K, Perren SM. Biology and biomechanics in bone healing. In: Ruedi TP, Buckley RE, Moran CG, eds. AO principles of fracture management. 2nd ed. Stuttgart: Thieme 2007; Vol 1: 8–31

Jäger M, Hernigou P, Zilkens C et al. Cell therapy in bone healing disorders. Orthop Rev (Pavia) 2010; 2: e20

Jagodzinski M, Krettek C. Effect of mechanical stability on fracture healing—an update. Injury 2007; 38 Suppl 1: S3–S10

Jehle M. Die Bedeutung des Vaso–Endothelialen Wachstumsfaktors (VEGF) in der Heilung von Frakturen unter Weichteilschaden und Schock (Dissertation). Medizinische Fakultät Uni Ulm; 2005

Jiang J, Papoutsakis ET. Stem-cell niche based comparative analysis of chemical and nano-mechanical material properties impacting ex vivo expansion and differentiation of hematopoietic and mesenchymal stem cells. Adv Healthc Mater 2013; 2: 25–42

Klein P, Schell H, Streitparth F et al. The initial phase of fracture healing is specifically sensitive to mechanical conditions. J Orthop Res 2003; 21: 662–669

Lacroix D, Prendergast PJ. A mechano-regulation model for tissue differentiation during fracture healing: analysis of gap size and loading. J Biomech 2002; 35: 1163–1171

Li S, Abdel-Wahab A, Silberschmidt VV. Analysis of fracture processes in cortical bone tissue. Eng Fract Mech 2013; 110: 448–458

Liedert A, Kaspar D, Blakytny R, Claes L, Ignatius A. Signal transduction pathways involved in mechanotransduction in bone cells. Biochem Biophys Res Commun 2006; 349: 1–5

McNamara LM, Prendergast PJ. Bone remodelling algorithms incorporating both strain and microdamage stimuli. J Biomech 2007; 40: 1381–1391

Morgan EF, Gleason RE, Hayward LN, Leong PL, Palomares KT. Mechanotransduction and fracture repair. J Bone Joint Surg Am 2008; 90 Suppl 1: 25–30

Morgan EF, Salisbury Palomares KT, Gleason RE et al. Correlations between local strains and tissue phenotypes in an experimental model of skeletal healing. J Biomech 2010; 43: 2418–2424

Ominsky MS, Li C, Li X et al. Inhibition of sclerostin by monoclonal antibody enhances bone healing and improves bone density and strength of nonfractured bones. J Bone Miner Res 2011; 26: 1012–1021

Palomares KT, Gleason RE, Mason ZD et al. Mechanical stimulation alters tissue differentiation and molecular expression during bone healing. J Orthop Res 2009; 27: 1123–1132

Perren SM. Fracture healing. The evolution of our understanding. Acta Chir Orthop Traumatol Cech 2008; 75: 241–246

Robling AG, Castillo AB, Turner CH. Biomechanical and molecular regulation of bone remodeling. Annu Rev Biomed Eng 2006; 8: 455–498

Santos A, Bakker AD, Klein-Nulend J. The role of osteocytes in bone mechanotransduction. Osteoporos Int 2009; 20: 1027–1031

Sathyendra V, Darowish M. Basic science of bone healing. Hand Clin 2013; 29: 473–481

Schell H, Epari DR, Kassi JP, Bragulla H, Bail HJ, Duda GN. The course of bone healing is influenced by the initial shear fixation stability. J Orthop Res 2005; 23: 1022–1028

Schmidt-Bleek K, Schell H, Schulz N et al. Inflammatory phase of bone healing initiates the regenerative healing cascade. Cell Tissue Res 2012; 347: 567–573

Seeman E. Bone modeling and remodeling. Crit Rev Eukaryot Gene Expr 2009; 19: 219–233

Thibault RA, Mikos AG, Kasper FK. Scaffold/Extracellular matrix hybrid constructs for bone-tissue engineering. Adv Healthc Mater 2013; 2: 13–24

Turner CH, Warden SJ, Bellido T et al. Mechanobiology of the skeleton. Sci Signal 2009; 2: pt3

Wehner T, Claes L, Niemeyer F, Nolte D, Simon U. Influence of the fixation stability on the healing time—a numerical study of a patient-specific fracture healing process. Clin Biomech (Bristol, Avon) 2010; 25: 606–612

11.3 Chapter 3: Non-operative Fracture Treatment

Al-Qattan MM, Al-Motairi MI, Al-Naeem HA. The diaphysial axis-metacarpal head angle in the management of fractures of the base of the proximal phalanx in children. J Hand Surg Eur Vol 2013; 38: 984–990

Barton N. Conservative treatment of articular fractures in the hand. J Hand Surg Am 1989; 14: 386–390

Burkhalter WE. Closed treatment of hand fractures. J Hand Surg Am 1989; 14: 390–393

Doornberg JN, Buijze GA, Ham SJ, Ring D, Bhandari M, Poolman RW. Nonoperative treatment for acute scaphoid fractures: a systematic review and meta-analysis of randomized controlled trials. J Trauma 2011; 71: 1073–1081

Ebinger T, Erhard N, Kinzl L, Mentzel M. Dynamic treatment of displaced proximal phalangeal fractures. J Hand Surg Am 199; 24: 1254–1262

Figl M, Wenninger P, HofbauerM, Pezzei Ch, Schauer J, Leixnering M. Results of Dynamic Treatment of Fractures of the Proximal Phalanx of the Hand. J Trauma-Injury Infection & Critical Care 2011; 70(4): 852–856

Franz T, Wartburg Uv, Hug U. Frühfunktionell-konservative Behandlung extraartikulärer Grundgliedfrakturen der Hand mit dem Luzerner Cast (LuCa)—Eine prospektive Pilotstudie. Handchir Mikrochir Plast Chir 2010; 42: 293–298

Freeland AE. Closed reduction of hand fractures. Clin Plast Surg 2005; 32: 549–561, vii

Giddins GEB. The non-operative management of hand fractures. J Hand Surg Eur Vol 2015; 40: 33–41

Hofmeister EP, Kim J, Shin AY. Comparison of 2 methods of immobilization of fifth metacarpal neck fractures: a prospective randomized study. J Hand Surg Am 2008; 33: 1362–1368

Hovgaard C, Klareskov B. Alternative conservative treatment of mallet-finger injuries by elastic double-finger bandage. J Hand Surg [Br] 1988; 13: 154–155

Janousek A, Zifko B, Klimesch E. Results of conservative treatment of bony palmar plate avulsion of the middle joint (type I and type II according to Hintringer and Leixnering). [Article in German.] Handchir Mikrochir Plast Chir 1996; 28: 242–245

Jehanno P, Mas V, Fitoussi J-M et al. Traumatismes osteoarticulaires des metacarpiens chez l'enfant. Chir Main 2013; 32: 29–38

Khan A, Giddins G. The outcome of conservative treatment of spiral metacarpal fractures and the role of the deep transverse metacarpal ligaments in stabilizing these injuries. J Hand Surg Eur Vol 2015; 40: 59–62

Kalainov DM, Hoepfner PE, Hartigan BJ, Carroll C, IV, Genuario J. Nonsurgical treatment of closed mallet finger fractures. J Hand Surg Am 2005; 30: 580–586

Kim JK, Kim DJ. The risk factors associated with subluxation of the distal interphalangeal joint in mallet fracture. J Hand Surg Eur Vol 2015; 40: 63–67

Leixnering M, Pezzei CH, Figl M. Funktionelle Behandlung von Grundgliedfrakturen. Zusammenfassungen- DAH 15.9.2005 www.dah.at/pdf/dah_abstracts05.pdf

Leixnering M. Versorgung von Problemfrakturen an Finger und Mittelhand. JATROS Unfallchirurgie und Sporttraumatologie 2009; 4: 8–11

Lubahn JD. Mallet finger fractures: a comparison of open and closed technique. J Hand Surg Am 1989; 14: 394–396

Pannier S, Dana C, Journe A et al. Les traumatismes distaux des doigts chez l'enfant Chir Main 2013; 32: 39–45

Pezzei C, Leixnering M, Hintringer W. Functional treatment of basal joint fractures of three-joint fingers. [Article in German.] Handchir Mikrochir Plast Chir 1993; 25: 319–329

Prokop A, Jubel A, Helling HJ, Kulus S, Rehm KE. Treatment of metacarpal fractures. [Article in German.] Handchir Mikrochir Plast Chir 2002; 34: 328–331

Puckett BN, Gaston RG, Peljovich AE, Lourie GM, Floyd WE, III. Remodeling potential of phalangeal distal condylar malunions in children. J Hand Surg Am 2012; 37: 34–41

Reiter A, Hasan M, Unglaub F, Dreyhaupt J, Hahn P. Conservative treatment results of the acute and chronic mallet finger. [Article in German.] Unfallchirurg 2005; 108: 1044–1048, 1046–1048

Sammer DM, Husain T, Ramirez R. Selection of appropriate treatment options for hand fractures. Hand Clin 2013; 29: 501–505

Schädel-Höpfner M, Lögters T, Windolf J, Gehrmann S, Eisenschenk A, Junge A. Current concepts in the treatment of mallet fractures of the distal phalanx. [Article in German.] Unfallchirurg 2011; 114: 591–596

, Sletten IN, Hellund JC, Olsen B, Clementsen S, Kvernmo HD, Nordsletten L. Conservative treatment has comparable outcome with bouquet pinning of little finger metacarpal neck fractures: a multicentre randomized controlled study of 85 patients. J Hand Surg Eur Vol 2015; 40: 76–83

Tang JB, Blazar PE, Giddins G, Lalonde D, Martínez C, Solomons M. Overview of indications, preferred methods and technical tips for hand fractures from around the world. J Hand Surg Eur Vol 2015; 40: 88–97

Thomine JM, Gibon Y, Bendjeddou MS, Biga N. Functional brace in the treatment of diaphyseal fractures of the proximal phalanges of the last four fingers. Ann Chir Main 1983; 2: 298–306

Weber P, Segmüller H. Non-surgical treatment of mallet finger fractures involving more than one third of the joint surface: 10 cases. [Article in German.] Handchir Mikrochir Plast Chir 2008; 40: 145–148

Wehbé MA, Schneider LH. Mallet fractures. J Bone Joint Surg Am 1984; 66: 658–669

11.4 Chapter 4: Surgical Fracture Management

Benjamin JFD, Little Ch. Fractures of the metacarpals and phalanges. Orthopaed Trauma 2011; 25: 43–56

Calfee RP, Sommerkamp TG. Fracture-dislocation about the finger joints. J Hand Surg Am 2009; 34: 1140–1147

Carpenter S, Rohde RS. Treatment of phalangeal fractures. Hand Clin 2013; 29: 519–534

Diaz-Garcia R, Waljee JF. Current management of metacarpal fractures. Hand Clin 2013; 29: 507–518

Ewerbeck V, Wentzensen A, Holz F, et al. Standardverfahren in der operativen Orthopädie und Unfallchirurgie. 3rd ed. Stuttgart: Thieme; 2007

Fitoussi F. Les fractures, luxations et entorses digitales chez l'enfant. Chir Main 2013; 32: S7–S15

Gajendran VK, Gajendran VK, Malone KJ. Management of complications with hand fractures. Hand Clin 2015; 31: 165–177

Haughton D, Jordan D, Malahias M, Hindocha S, Khan W. Principles of hand fracture management. Open Orthop J 2012; 6: 43–53

Heim U, Pfeiffer KM. Periphere Osteosynthesen. 4. Auflge. Berlin: Springer; 1991

Hoffmann R. Checkliste Handchirurgie Stuttgart: Thieme; 1997

Jones NF, Jupiter JB, Lalonde DH. Common fractures and dislocations of the hand. Plast Reconstr Surg 2012; 130: 722e–736e

Jupiter J, Ring D. AO manual of fracture management: Hand and wrist. Stuttgart: Thieme; 2005

Kremer K, Lierse W, Platzer W, et al. Chirurgische Operationslehre. Schultergurtel, obere Extremität, Hand, Finger. Stuttgart: Thieme; 1995

Lawson E, Thomsen L, Hans-Moevi Akué A, Falcone MO. Complex fracture-dislocation of the proximal interphalangeal joint. A case report and focus on palmar proximal interphalangeal fractures-dislocations. [Article in French.] Chir Main 2013; 32: 28: 1–286

Leixnering M. Versorgung von Problemfrakturen an Finger und Mittelhand. JATROS Unfallchirurgie und Sporttraumatologie 2009; 4: 8–10

Liodaki E, Xing SG, Mailaender P, Stang F. Management of difficult intra-articular fractures or fracture dislocations of the proximal interphalangeal joint. J Hand Surg Eur Vol 2015; 40: 16–23

Liverneaux PA, Ichihara S, Hendriks S, Facca S, Bodin F. Fractures and dislocation of the base of the thumb metacarpal. J Hand Surg Eur Vol 2015; 40: 42–50

Martini A-K. Orthopädie und Orthopädische Chirurgie. Stuttgart: Thieme; 2003

Merle M, Voche P. Chirurgie der Hand. Stuttgart: Thieme; 2012

Müller MC, Ekkernkamp A, Frakturen. Heidelberg: Springer; 2010

Müller ME, Allgöwer M, Schneider R, et al. Manual der Osteosynthese. 3. Auflage. Berlin: Springer; 1992

Nellans KW, Chung KC. Pediatric hand fractures. Hand Clin 2013; 29: 569–578

Nigst H, Buck-Gramcko D, Millesi H. Handchirurgie. Band II. Stuttgart: Thieme; 1983

Nigst H, Haussmann P. 10 Gebote des atraumatischen Operierens. Mündliche Mitteilung

Nigst H, Hrsg. Frakturen der Hand und des Handgelenkes Stuttgart: Hippokrates; 1988

Oak N, Lawton JN. Intra-articular fractures of the hand. Hand Clin 2013; 29: 535–549

Osteosynthese am Handskelett. Stuttgart: Thieme OP-Journal 1991; 2(7)

Pechlaner S, Hussl H, Kerschbaumer F. Operationsatlas Handchirurgie. Stuttgart: Thieme; 1998

Pegoli L, Badia A, Bain G et al. IFSSH Sport Committee Report IFSSH ezine; Nov 2013: 19–28

Rudigier J. Kurzgefasste Handchirurgie. 4. Auflage. Stuttgart: Thieme; 2006

Schädel-Höpfner M, Prommersberger KJ, Eisenschenk A, Windolf J. Treatment of carpal fractures. Recommendations of the Hand Surgery Group of the German Trauma Society. [Article in German.] Unfallchirurg 2010; 113: 741–754, quiz 755

Schaefer M, Siebert HR. Finger and metacarpal fractures. Surgical and non-surgical treatment procedures. I. [Article in German.] Unfallchirurg 2000; 103: 482–494

Schaefer M, Siebert HR. Finger and middle hand fractures. Surgical and non-surgical treatment procedures. II. [Article in German.] Unfallchirurg 2000; 103: 582–592

Shah CM, Sommerkamp TG. Fracture dislocation of the finger joints. J Hand Surg Am 2014; 39: 792–802

Shewring DJ, Miller AC, Ghandour A. Condylar fractures of the proximal and middle phalanges. J Hand Surg Eur Vol 2015; 40: 51–58

Stern PJ. Management of fractures of the hand over the last 25 years. J Hand Surg Am 2000; 25: 817–823

Tsuge K. Atlas der Handchirurgie. Stuttgart: Hippokrates; 1991

Watanabe K, Kino Y, Yajima H. Factors affecting the functional results of open reduction and internal fixation for fracture-dislocations of the proximal interphalangeal joint. Hand Surg 2015; 20: 107–114

Wada T, Oda T. Mallet fingers with bone avulsion and DIP joint subluxation. J Hand Surg Eur Vol 2015; 40: 8–15

Windolf J, Rueger JM, Werber KD, Eisenschenk A, Siebert H, Schädel-Höpfner M. Treatment of metacarpal fractures. Recommendations of the Hand Surgery Group of the German Trauma Society. [Article in German.] Unfallchirurg 2009; 112: 577–588, quiz 589

Windolf J, Siebert H, Werber KD, Schädel-Höpfner M. Treatment of phalangeal fractures: recommendations of the Hand Surgery Group of the German Trauma Society. [Article in German.] Unfallchirurg 2008; 111: 331–338, quiz 339

Zach A, Lautenbacher M, Merk H et al. Frakturen der Phalangen Handchirurgie Scan 2013; 1: 49–65

11.5 Chapter 5: Differential Indication

Petracić B, Siebert H. AO-classification of fractures of the hand bones. [Article in German.] Handchir Mikrochir Plast Chir 1998; 30: 40–44

11.6 Chapter 7: Postoperative Management

Bonten A. Kern p. Therapierichtlinien der Nachbehandlung nach Frakturen der Mittelhand. OP-Journal 1991; 2: 83–86

Bureck W. Aims of hand therapy in treatment of rheumatoid hand. [Article in German.] Handchir Mikrochir Plast Chir 2005; 37: 52–59

Feehan LM, Tang CS, Oxland TR. Early controlled passive motion improves early fracture alignment and structural properties in a closed extra-articular metacarpal fracture in a rabbit model. J Hand Surg Am 2007; 32: 200–208

Freeland AE, Hardy MA, Singletary S. Rehabilitation for proximal phalangeal fractures. J Hand Ther 2003; 16: 129–142

Freeland AE, Orbay JL. Extraarticular hand fractures in adults: a review of new developments. Clin Orthop Relat Res 2006; 445: 133–145

, Guzelkucuk U, Duman I, Taskaynatan MA, Dincer K. Comparison of therapeutic activities with therapeutic exercises in the rehabilitation of young adult patients with hand injuries. J Hand Surg Am 2007; 32: 1429: 1435

Haarer-Becker R, Schoer D. Physiotherapie in Orthopädie und Traumatologie. Stuttgart: Thieme; 1996

Holzer K. Occupational therapy after rheumatoid hand surgery. [Article in German.] Handchir Mikrochir Plast Chir 2005; 37: 60–66

Lowka K. Nachbehandlung nach Osteosynthesen am Handskelett. OP-Journal 1991; 2: 73–82

Nigst H. Ergo-, Physio- und Physikotherpie. In: Nigst H, Buck-Gramcko D, Milesi H, Hrsg. Handchirurgie. Band I. Stuttgart: Thieme; 1981

Schröder B. Handtherapie. Stuttgart: Thieme; 2008

Waldner-Nilsson B. Ergotherapie in der Handrehabilitation. Band I und II. 2. Auflage. Berlin: Springer; 2009

11.7 Chapter 8: Implants and Instruments

Mudgal CS, Jupiter JB. Plate and screw design in fractures of the hand and wrist. Clin Orthop Relat Res 2006; 445: 68–80

11.8 Chapter 9: Surgical Approaches

AO Foundation. Surgical References—Hand Approaches. Im Internet: https://www2.aofoundation.org/wps/portal/surgery; Accessed: 04.02.2013

Berger RA. A method of defining palpable landmarks for the ligament-splitting dorsal wrist capsulotomy. J Hand Surg Am 2007; 32: 1291–1295

Cardoso R, Szabo RM. Wrist anatomy and surgical approaches. Hand Clin 2010; 26: 1–19

Catalano LW, Zlotolow DA, Purcelli Lafer M, Weidner Z, Barron OA. Surgical exposures of the wrist and hand. J Am Acad Orthop Surg 2012; 20: 48–57

Ewerbeck V, Wentzensen A. Standardverfahren in der operativen Orthopädie und Unfallchirurgie. 3. Auflage. Stuttgart: Thieme; 2007

Garcia-Elias M, Hagert E. Surgical approaches to the distal radioulnar joint. Hand Clin 2010; 26: 477–483

Hagert E, Ferreres A, Garcia-Elias M. Nerve-sparing dorsal and volar approaches to the radiocarpal joint. J Hand Surg Am 2010; 35: 1070–1074

Henry M. Soft tissue sleeve approach to open reduction and internal fixation of proximal phalangeal fractures. Tech Hand Up Extrem Surg 2008; 12: 161–165

Koebke J. Operative Zugänge nach funktionell—anatomischen Gesichtspunkten. OP-Journal 1991; 2: 8–11

Pechlaner S, Kerschbaumer F, Hussl H. Operationsatlas Handchirurgie. Stuttgart: Thieme; 1998

Schmidt HM, Lanz U. Chirurgische Anatomie der Hand. Stuttgart: Thieme; 1992

Tay SC, Shin AY. Surgical approaches to the carpus. Hand Clin 2006; 22: 421–434, abstract v

Tubiana R, McCullough CJ, Masquelet AC. Atlas der operativen Zugangswege Schultergürtel und obere Extremität. Köln: Deutscher Ärzte Verlag; 1992 von Torklus HD. Atlas orthopadisch–chirurgischer Zugangswege. 3. Auflage. München: Urban & Schwarzenberg; 1992

Wei DH, Strauch RJ. Dorsal surgical approaches to the proximal interphalangeal joint: a comparative anatomic study. J Hand Surg Am 2014; 39: 1082–1087

11.9 Chapter 10: Surgical Procedures

11.9.1 Wire Suture, Tension Band Wiring

Adler H. Tension band osteosynthesis in osseous finger extensor tendon rupture (so-called Bush fracture). [Article in German,] Handchir Mikrochir Plast Chir 1982; 14: 121–122

Al-Qattan MM. Metacarpal shaft fractures of the fingers: treatment with interosseous loop wire fixation and immediate postoperative finger mobilisation in a wrist splint. J Hand Surg [Br] 2006; 31: 377–382

Bischoff R, Buechler U, De Roche R, Jupiter J. Clinical results of tension band fixation of avulsion fractures of the hand. J Hand Surg Am 1994; 19: 1019–1026

Brüser P. Drahtnahtosteosynthesen an der Hand. In: Nigst H, Hrsg. Frakturen der Hand und des Handgelenkes. Stuttgart: Hippokrates; 1988

Jupiter JB, Sheppard JE. Tension wire fixation of avulsion fractures in the hand. Clin Orthop Relat Res 1987: 113–120

Kamath JB, Vardhan H, Naik DM, Bharadwaj P, Menezes RJ, Sayoojianadhan BP. Modified bone tie: a new method to achieve interfragmentary compression in unstable oblique metacarpal and phalangeal fractures. Tech Hand Up Extrem Surg 2012; 16: 42–44

Kozin SH, Bishop AT. Tension wire fixation of avulsion fractures at the thumb metacarpophalangeal joint. J Hand Surg Am 1994; 19: 1027–1031

Lee H-J, Jeon I-H, Kim P-T, Oh CW, Deslivia MF, Lee SJ. Transtendinous wiring of mallet finger fractures presenting late. J Hand Surg Am 2014; 39: 2383–2389

Narr H, Reill P. Die Behandlung des knöchernen Strecksehnenabrisses. Plast Chir 1980; 4: 102–107

11.9.2 Lag Screw, Plate Fixation

Afshar R, Fong TS, Latifi MH, Kanthan SR, Kamarul T. A biomechanical study comparing plate fixation using unicortical and bicortical screws in transverse metacarpal fracture models subjected to cyclic loading. J Hand Surg Eur Vol 2012; 37: 396–401

Bannasch H, Heermann AK, Iblher N, Momeni A, Schulte-Mönting J, Stark GB. Ten years stable internal fixation of metacarpal and phalangeal hand fractures—risk factor and outcome analysis show no increase of complications in the treatment of open compared with closed fractures. J Trauma 2010; 68: 624–628

Bartelmann U, Müller O, Kalb K, Landsleitner B. Is mini-screw osteosynthesis a suitable procedure in surgical treatment of intra-articular distal phalanx fractures? [Article in German.] Handchir Mikrochir Plast Chir 2001; 33: 41–45

Chim H, Teoh LC, Yong FC. Open reduction and interfragmentary screw fixation for symptomatic nonunion of distal phalangeal fractures. J Hand Surg Eur Vol 2008; 33: 71–76

Dabezies EJ, Schutte JP. Fixation of metacarpal and phalangeal fractures with miniature plates and screws. J Hand Surg Am 1986; 11: 283–288

Dean BJF, Little C. Fractures of the metacarpals and phalanges. Orthop Trauma 2011; 25: 43–56

Diao E, Welborn JH. Extraarticular fractures of the metacarpals. In: Berger AR, Weiss A-PC, eds. Hand Surgery. Philadelphia: Lippincott Williams & Wilkins; 2004

Dona E, Gillies RM, Gianoutsos MP, Walsh WR. Plating of metacarpal fractures: unicortical or bicortical screws? J Hand Surg [Br] 2004; 29: 218–221

Freeland AE, Orbay JL. Extraarticular hand fractures in adults: a review of new developments. Clin Orthop Relat Res 2006; 445: 133–145

Freeland AE, Sud V. Unicondylar and bicondylar proximal phalangeal fractures. J Am Soc Surg Hand 2001; 1: 14–24

Fufa DT, Goldfarb CA. Fractures of the thumb and finger metacarpals in athletes. Hand Clin 2012; 28: 379–388, x

Gaston RG, Chadderdon C. Phalangeal fractures: displaced/nondisplaced. Hand Clin 2012; 28: 395–401, x

Grant I, Berger AC, Tham SK. Internal fixation of unstable fracture dislocations of the proximal interphalangeal joint. J Hand Surg [Br] 2005; 30: 492–498

Hamilton SC, Stern PJ, Fassler PR, Kiefhaber TR. Mini-screw fixation for the treatment of proximal interphalangeal joint dorsal fracture-dislocations. J Hand Surg Am 2006; 31: 1349–1354

Hattori Y, Doi K, Sakamoto S, Yamasaki H, Wahegaonkar A, Addosooki A. Volar plating for intra-articular fracture of the base of the proximal phalanx. J Hand Surg Am 2007; 32: 1299–1303

Heermann AK. Retrospektive Untersuchung bewegungsstabiler Schrauben- und Plattenosteosythesen an Mittelhand und Finger (Dissertation). Universität Freiburg; 2005

Henry MH. Fractures of the proximal phalanx and metacarpals in the hand: preferred methods of stabilization. J Am Acad Orthop Surg 2008; 16: 586–595

Khalid M, Theivendran K, Cheema M, Rajaratnam V, Deshmukh SC. Biomechanical comparison of pull-out force of unicortical versus bicortical screws in proximal phalanges of the hand: a human cadaveric study. Clin Biomech (Bristol, Avon) 2008; 23: 1136–1140

Karadeniz E, Balcik BC, Demirors H, Tuncay IC. Biomechanical comparison of conventional technique versus oblique screw placement in plate fixation. J Trauma 2011; 70: E84–E87

Lee JYL, Teoh LC. Dorsal fracture dislocations of the proximal interphalangeal joint treated by open reduction and interfragmentary screw fixation: indications, approaches and results. J Hand Surg [Br] 2006; 31: 138–146

Nicklin S, Ingram S, Gianoutsos MP, Walsh WR. In vitro comparison of lagged and nonlagged screw fixation of metacarpal fractures in cadavers. J Hand Surg Am 2008; 33: 1732–1736

Omokawa S, Fujitani R, Dohi Y, Okawa T, Yajima H. Prospective outcomes of comminuted periarticular metacarpal and phalangeal fractures treated using a titanium plate system. J Hand Surg Am 2008; 33: 857–863

del Piñal F, Moraleda E, Rúas JS, de Piero GH, Cerezal L. Minimally invasive fixation of fractures of the phalanges and metacarpals with intramedullary cannulated headless compression screws. J Hand Surg Am 2015; 40: 692–700

Prevel CD, Eppley BL, Jackson RJ et al. Mini and micro plating of phalangeal and metacarpal fractures: a biomechanical study. J Hand Surg Am 1995; 20: 44–49

Roth JJ, Auerbach DM. Fixation of hand fractures with bicortical screws. J Hand Surg Am 2005; 30: 151–153

Ruchelsman DE, Puri S, Feinberg-Zadek N, Leibman MI, Belsky MR. Clinical outcomes of limited-open retrograde intramedullary headless screw fixation of metacarpal fractures. J Hand Surg Am 2014; 39: 2390–2395

Rudigier J. Kurzgefasste Handchirurgie. 4. Auflage. Stuttgart:Thieme; 2006

Schädel–Höpfner M, Windolf J. Hand. In: Müller-Mai CM, Ekkernkamp A, Hrsg. Frakturen. Heidelberg: Springer; 2010

Sohn RC, Jahng KH, Curtiss SB, Szabo RM. Comparison of metacarpal plating methods. J Hand Surg Am 2008; 33: 316–321

Soni A, Gulati A, Bassi JL, Singh D, Saini UC. Outcome of closed ipsilateral metacarpal fractures treated with mini fragment plates and screws: a prospective study. J Orthop Traumatol 2012; 13: 29–33

Souer JS, Mudgal CS. Plate fixation in closed ipsilateral multiple metacarpal fractures. J Hand Surg Eur Vol 2008; 33: 740–744

Strassmair M, Wilhelm K. Verletzungen und Verletzungsfolgen im Handgelenkbereich.In: Martini AK. Ellenbogen, Unterarm, Hand. In: Wirth CJ, Zichner L (Reihen Hrsg). Orthopädie und orthopädische Chirurgie. Thieme: Stuttgart, New York; 2003

Van Schoonhoven J, Stang F, Prommersberger KJ. Bone Injury. Curr Orthop 2008; 22: 25–30

Williams CS, IV. Proximal interphalangeal joint fracture dislocations: stable and unstable. Hand Clin 2012; 28: 409–416, xi

Windolf J, Rueger JM, Werber KD, Eisenschenk A, Siebert H, Schädel-Höpfner M. Treatment of metacarpal fractures. Recommendations of the Hand Surgery Group of the German Trauma Society. [Article in German.] Unfallchirurg 2009; 112: 577–588, quiz 589

, Windolf J, Siebert H, Werber KD, Schädel-Höpfner M. Treatment of phalangeal fractures: recommendations of the Hand Surgery Group of the German Trauma Society. [Article in German.] Unfallchirurg 2008; 111: 331–338, quiz 339

Wong HC, Lam C, Wong KY et al. Treatment of phalangeal and metacarpal fractures: a review. Pb J Orthop 2008; X: 42–50

Wong KP, Hay RAS, Tay SC. Surgical outcomes of fifth metacarpal neck fractures—a comparative analysis of dorsal plating versus tension band wiring. Hand Surg 2015; 20: 99–105

11.9.3 Fixed-angle Locking Plate

Aguila AZ, Manos JM, Orlansky AS, Todhunter RJ, Trotter EJ, Van der Meulen MC. In vitro biomechanical comparison of limited contact dynamic compression plate and locking compression plate. Vet Comp Orthop Traumatol 2005; 18: 220–226

Ahmad M, Nanda R, Bajwa AS, Candal-Couto J, Green S, Hui AC. Biomechanical testing of the locking compression plate: when does the distance between bone and implant significantly reduce construct stability? Injury 2007; 38: 358–364

Barr C, Behn AW, Yao J. Plating of metacarpal fractures with locked or nonlocked screws, a biomechanical study: how many cortices are really necessary? Hand (NY) 2013; 8: 454–459

Claes L. Biomechanical principles and mechanobiologic aspects of flexible and locked plating. J Orthop Trauma 2011; 25 Suppl 1: S4–S7

Cullen AB, Curtiss S, Lee MA. Biomechanical comparison of polyaxial and uniaxial locking plate fixation in a proximal tibial gap model. J Orthop Trauma 2009; 23: 507–513

Denard PJ, Doornink J, Phelan D, Madey SM, Fitzpatrick DC, Bottlang M. Biplanar fixation of a locking plate in the diaphysis improves construct strength. Clin Biomech (Bristol, Avon) 2011; 26: 484–490

Diaconu M, Facca S, Gouzou S, Liverneaux P. Locking plates for fixation of extra-articular fractures of the first metacarpal base: a series of 15 cases. Chir Main 2011; 30: 26–30

Doht S, Jansen H, Meffert R, Frey S. Higher stability with locking plates in hand surgery? Biomechanical investigation of the TriLock system in a fracture model. Int Orthop 2012; 36: 1641–1646

Doornink J, Fitzpatrick DC, Madey SM, Bottlang M. Far cortical locking enables flexible fixation with periarticular locking plates. J Orthop Trauma 2011; 25 Suppl 1: S29–S34

Eichinger JK, Herzog JP, Arrington ED. Analysis of the mechanical properties of locking plates with and without screw hole inserts. Orthopedics 2011; 34: 19

Facca S, Ramdhian R, Pelissier A, Diaconu M, Liverneaux P. Fifth metacarpal neck fracture fixation: Locking plate versus K-wire? Orthop Traumatol Surg Res 2010; 96: 506–512

Gajendran VK, Szabo RM, Myo GK, Curtiss SB. Biomechanical comparison of double-row locking plates versus single- and double-row non-locking plates in a comminuted metacarpal fracture model. J Hand Surg Am 2009; 34: 1851–1858

Gardner MJ, Evans JM, Dunbar RP. Failure of fracture plate fixation. J Am Acad Orthop Surg 2009; 17: 647–657

Garrigues GE, Glisson RR, Garrigues NW, Richard MJ, Ruch DS. Can locking screws allow smaller, low-profile plates to achieve comparable stability to larger, standard plates? J Orthop Trauma 2011; 25: 347–354

Gautier E, Sommer C. Guidelines for the clinical application of the LCP. Injury 2003; 34 Suppl 2: B63–B76

Gebhard C. Biomechanischer Stabilitätsvergleich zwei- und dreidimensionaler, winkelstabiler Miniimplantate für die Osteosynthese von Mittelhandfrakturen (Dissertation). Universität Würzburg; 2010

Kubiak EN, Fulkerson E, Strauss E, Egol KA. The evolution of locked plates. J Bone Joint Surg Am 2006; 88 Suppl 4: 189–200

Larson AN, Rizzo M. Locking plate technology and its applications in upper extremity fracture care. Hand Clin 2007; 23: 269–278, vii

Lautenbach M, Zach A, Eisenschenk A. Winkelstabile Implantate an der Hand. Trauma Berufskrankheit 2012; 14 Suppl. 2: 164–170

Liodaki E, Schopp BE, Wendtlandt R et al. Ist weniger mehr? Monokortikale vs. bikortikale Osteosynthese von Mittelhandfrakturen—eine biomechanische Studie. 2014 Vortrag Sept 2014 München, Open Accesss article doi: 10.3205/14dgpraec238

Miller DL, Goswami T. A review of locking compression plate biomechanics and their advantages as internal fixators in fracture healing. Clin Biomech (Bristol, Avon) 2007; 22: 1049–1062

Niemeyer P, Sudkamp NP. Principles and clinical application of the locking compression plate (LCP). Acta Chir Orthop Traumatol Cech 2006; 73: 221–228

Ochman S, Doht S, Paletta J, Langer M, Raschke MJ, Meffert RH. Comparison between locking and non-locking plates for fixation of metacarpal fractures in an animal model. J Hand Surg Am 2010; 35: 597–603

Oh JK, Sahu D, Ahn YH et al. Effect of fracture gap on stability of compression plate fixation: a finite element study. J Orthop Res 2010; 28: 462–467

Ruchelsman DE, Mudgal CS, Jupiter JB. The role of locking technology in the hand. Hand Clin 2010; 26: 307–319, v

Snow M, Thompson G, Turner PG. A mechanical comparison of the locking compression plate (LCP) and the low contact-dynamic compression plate (DCP) in an osteoporotic bone model. J Orthop Trauma 2008; 22: 121–125

Stoffel K, Dieter U, Stachowiak G, Gächter A, Kuster MS. Biomechanical testing of the LCP—how can stability in locked internal fixators be controlled? Injury 2003; 34 Suppl 2: B11–B19

Strauss EJ, Schwarzkopf R, Kummer F, Egol KA. The current status of locked plating: the good, the bad, and the ugly. J Orthop Trauma 2008; 22: 479–486

Tan SL, Balogh ZJ. Indications and limitations of locked plating. Injury 2009; 40: 683–691

Windolf M, Klos K, Wähnert D et al. Biomechanical investigation of an alternative concept to angular stable plating using conventional fixation hardware. BMC Musculoskelet Disord 2010; 11: 95–99

Wong HC, Wong HK, Wong KY. Stainless steel 2.0-mm locking compression plate osteosynthesis system for the fixation of comminuted hand fractures in Asian adults. J Orthop Trauma Reha 2011; 15: 57–61

Ya'ish FM, Nanu AM, Cross AT. Can DCP and LCP plates generate more compression? The effect of multiple eccentrically placed screws and their drill positioning guides. Injury 2011; 42: 1095–1100

Yaffe MA, Saucedo JM, Kalainov DM. Non-locked and locked plating technology for hand fractures. J Hand Surg Am 2011; 36: 2052–2055

11.9.4 Hybrid Plate

Bottlang M, Doornink J, Byrd GD, Fitzpatrick DC, Madey SM. A nonlocking end screw can decrease fracture risk caused by locked plating in the osteoporotic diaphysis. J Bone Joint Surg Am 2009; 91: 620–627

Doornink J, Fitzpatrick DC, Boldhaus S, Madey SM, Bottlang M. Effects of hybrid plating with locked and nonlocked screws on the strength of locked plating constructs in the osteoporotic diaphysis. J Trauma 2010; 69: 411–417

Dunlap JT, Lucas GL, Chong AC, Cooke FW, Tiruvadi V. Biomechanical evaluation of locking plate fixation with hybrid screw constructs in analogue humeri. Am J Orthop 2011; 40: E20–E25

Lujan TJ, Henderson CE, Madey SM, Fitzpatrick DC, Marsh JL, Bottlang M. Locked plating of distal femur fractures leads to inconsistent and asymmetric callus formation. J Orthop Trauma 2010; 24: 156–162

Roberts JW, Grindel SI, Rebholz B, Wang M. Biomechanical evaluation of locking plate radial shaft fixation: unicortical locking fixation versus mixed bicortical and unicortical fixation in a sawbone model. J Hand Surg Am 2007; 32: 971–975

Stoffel K, Lorenz K-U, Kuster MS. Biomechanical considerations in plate osteosynthesis: the effect of plate-to-bone compression with and without angular screw stability. J Orthop Trauma 2007; 21: 362–368

Sutherland GB, Creekmore T, Mukherjee DP, Ogden AL, Anissian L, Marymont JV. Biomechanics of humerus fracture fixation by locking, cortical, and hybrid plating systems in a cadaver model. Orthopedics 2010; 33: 8

Wagner M. General principles for the clinical use of the LCP. Injury 2003; 34 Suppl 2: B31–B42

11.9.5 Condylar Plate

Büchler U. Mini condylar plate osteosyntheses of the hand. [Article in German.] Handchir Mikrochir Plast Chir 1987; 19: 136–144

Büchler U, Fischer T. Use of a minicondylar plate for metacarpal and phalangeal periarticular injuries. Clin Orthop Relat Res 1987: 53–58

11.9.6 Far locking / Dynamic Screw Technique

Bottlang M, Doornink J, Fitzpatrick DC, Madey SM. Far cortical locking can reduce stiffness of locked plating constructs while retaining construct strength. J Bone Joint Surg Am 2009; 91: 1985–1994

Bottlang M, Doornink J, Lujan TJ et al. Effects of construct stiffness on healing of fractures stabilized with locking plates. J Bone Joint Surg Am 2010; 92 Suppl 2: 12–22

Bottlang M, Feist F. Biomechanics of far cortical locking. J Orthop Trauma 2011; 25: 21–28

Bottlang M, Lesser M, Koerber J et al. Far cortical locking can improve healing of fractures stabilized with locking plates. J Bone Joint Surg Am 2010; 92: 1652–1660

Döbele S, Horn C, Eichhorn S et al. The dynamic locking screw (DLS) can increase interfragmentary motion on the near cortex of locked plating constructs by reducing the axial stiffness. Langenbecks Arch Surg 2010; 395: 421–428

Gardner MJ, Nork SE, Huber P, Krieg JC. Less rigid stable fracture fixation in osteoporotic bone using locked plates with near cortical slots. Injury 2010; 41: 652–656

Sellei RM, Garrison RL, Kobbe P, Lichte P, Knobe M, Pape HC. Effects of near cortical slotted holes in locking plate constructs. J Orthop Trauma 2011; 25 Suppl 1: S35–S40

11.9.7 Headless Bone Screw (HBS)

Carpal Bones

Botte MJ, Gelberman RH. Fractures of the carpus, excluding the scaphoid. Hand Clin 1987; 3: 149–161

Cohen MS. Fractures of the carpal bones. Hand Clin 1997; 13: 587–599

Garcia-Elias M, Mathoulin ChL. 2014

Gardner AW, Yew YT, Neo PY, Lau CC, Tay SC. Interfragmentary compression profile of 4 headless bone screws: an analysis of the compression lost on reinsertion. J Hand Surg Am 2012; 37: 1845–1851

Journeau P.. Traumatismes du carpe chez l'enfant. Chirurgie de la Main 2013; 32: 16–28

Moritomo H, Aspergis E, Herzberg G et al.. Committee Report on wrist biomechanics and instability: Carpal instability following scaphoid fracture. IFSSH ezine 2011; 4: 14–17

Schädel-Höpfner M, Prommersberger KJ, Eisenschenk A, Windolf J. Treatment of carpal fractures. Recommendations of the Hand Surgery Group of the German Trauma Society. [Article in German.] Unfallchirurg 2010; 113: 741–754, quiz 755

Suh N, Ek ET, Wolfe SW. Carpal fractures. J Hand Surg Am 2014; 39: 785–791, quiz 791

Vigler M, Aviles A, Lee SK. Carpal fractures excluding the scaphoid. Hand Clin 2006; 22: 501–516, abstract vii

Scaphoid Bone

Arora R, Gschwentner M, Krappinger D, Lutz M, Blauth M, Gabl M. Fixation of nondisplaced scaphoid fractures: making treatment cost effective. Prospective controlled trial. Arch Orthop Trauma Surg 2007; 127: 39–46

Bedi A, Jebson PJL, Hayden RJ, Jacobson JA, Martus JE. Internal fixation of acute, nondisplaced scaphoid waist fractures via a limited dorsal approach: an assessment of radiographic and functional outcomes. J Hand Surg Am 2007; 32: 326–333

Bushnell BD, McWilliams AD, Messer TM. Complications in dorsal percutaneous cannulated screw fixation of nondisplaced scaphoid waist fractures. J Hand Surg Am 2007; 32: 827–833

Doornberg JN, Buijze GA, Ham SJ, Ring D, Bhandari M, Poolman RW. Nonoperative treatment for acute scaphoid fractures: a systematic review and meta-analysis of randomized controlled trials. J Trauma 2011; 71: 1073–1081

Herbert TJ, Fisher WE. Management of the fractured scaphoid using a new bone screw. J Bone Joint Surg Br 1984; 66: 114–123

Herbert TJ. Internal fixation of the carpus with the Herbert bone screw system. J Hand Surg Am 1989; 14: 397–400

Ibrahim T, Qureshi A, Sutton AJ, Dias JJ. Surgical versus nonsurgical treatment of acute minimally displaced and undisplaced scaphoid waist fractures: pairwise and network meta-analyses of randomized controlled trials. J Hand Surg Am 2011; 36: 1759–1768.e1

Karle B, Mayer B, Kitzinger HB, Fröhner S, Schmitt R, Krimmer H. Scaphoid fractures—operative or conservative treatment? A CT-based classification. [Article in German.] Handchir Mikrochir Plast Chir 2005; 37: 260–266

Kraus R, Böhringer G, Meyer C, Stahl JP, Schnettler R. Fractures of the scaphoid tubercle. [Article in German.] Handchir Mikrochir Plast Chir 2005; 37: 79–84

Krimmer H. Kahnbeinfraktur—Diagnostik und Therapie—aktueller Stand. Obere Extremität 2010; 5: 98–105

Luria S, Hoch S, Liebergall M, Mosheiff R, Peleg E. Optimal fixation of acute scaphoid fractures: finite element analysis. J Hand Surg Am 2010; 35: 1246–1250

Preisser P, Rudolf KD, Partecke BD. Surgical treatment of scaphoid pseudarthrosis—long term outcome with the Herbert screws. [Article in German.] Handchir Mikrochir Plast Chir 1998; 30: 45–51

Sauerbier M, German G. Skaphoidfraktur. In: Ewerbeck V, Wentzensen A, Hrsg. Standardverfahren in der operativen Orthopädie und Unfallchirurgie. 3. Auflage. Stuttgart: Thieme; 2007

Schädel-Höpfner M, Böhringer G, Gotzen L. Percutaneous osteosynthesis of scaphoid fracture with the Herbert-Whipple screw—technique and results. [Article in German.] Handchir Mikrochir Plast Chir 2000; 32: 271–276

Triquetral Bone

Kessler T, Köpke J, Gebert L. Simultaneous corpus fractures of the os triquetrum and os hamatum diagnosed by magnetic resonance tomography. A case report. [Article in German.] Handchir Mikrochir Plast Chir 1996; 28: 50–52

Scharizer E. Die Verletzung des Os triquetrum. In: Nigst H, Hrsg. Frakturen, Luxationen und Dissoziationen der Karpalknochen. Stuttgart: Hippokrates; 1982

Suzuki T, Nakatsuchi Y, Tateiwa Y, Tsukada A, Yotsumoto N. Osteochondral fracture of the triquetrum: a case report. J Hand Surg Am 2002; 27: 98–100

Lunate Bone

Höcker K, Renner J. Fracture of the lunate—a rare injury. [Article in German.] Handchir Mikrochir Plast Chir 1995; 27: 247–253

Scharizer E. Die Verletzungen des Os lunatum. In: Nigst H, Hrsg. Frakturen, Luxationen und Dissoziationen der Karpalknochen. Stuttgart: Hippokrates; 1982

Trapezium

Binhammer P, Born T. Coronal fracture of the body of the trapezium: a case report. J Hand Surg Am 1998; 23: 156–157

Freeland AE, Finley JS. Displaced vertical fracture of the trapezium treated with a small cancellous lag screw. J Hand Surg Am 1984; 9: 843–845

Jones JA, Pellegrini VD, Jr. Transverse fracture-dislocation of the trapezium. J Hand Surg Am 1989; 14: 481–485

McGuigan FX, Culp RW. Surgical treatment of intra-articular fractures of the trapezium. J Hand Surg Am 2002; 27: 697–703

Trapezoid Bone

Kain N, Heras-Palou C. Trapezoid fractures: report of 11 cases. J Hand Surg Am 2012; 37: 1159–1162

Capitate Bone

Apergis E, Darmanis S, Kastanis G, Papanikolaou A. Does the term scaphocapitate syndrome need to be revised? A report of 6 cases. J Hand Surg [Br] 2001; 26: 441–445

Arbter D, Piatek S, Wichlas F, Winckler S. The scaphocapitate fracture syndrome (Fenton). [Article in German.] Handchir Mikrochir Plast Chir 2009; 41: 171–174

D'Hondt B, Safi A, Brüser P. Die Pseudarthrose des Os capitatum. Bericht über zwei Fälle. Handchir Mikrochir Plast Chir 1997; 29: 27–31

Fenton RL. The naviculo-capitate fracture syndrome. J Bone Joint Surg Am 1956; 38-A: 681–684

Gehrmann SV, Wild M, Windolf J, Hakimi MY. Isolated fractures of the capitate: treatment of delayed union. [Article in German.] Handchir Mikrochir Plast Chir 2009; 41: 175–178

Klitscher D, Hückstädt T, Müller LP, Weltzien A, Schier F, Rommens PM. Capitate fracture in an 11-year-old boy. [Article in German.] Handchir Mikrochir Plast Chir 2010; 42: 314–316

Hamate Bone

Bishop AT, Beckenbaugh RD. Fracture of the hamate hook. J Hand Surg Am 1988; 13: 135–139

Bowen TL. Injuries of the hamate bone. Hand 1973; 5: 235–238

Kimura H, Kamura S, Akai M, Ohno T. An unusual coronal fracture of the body of the hamate bone. J Hand Surg Am 1988; 13: 743–745

Loth TS, McMillan MD. Coronal dorsal hamate fractures. J Hand Surg Am 1988; 13: 616–618

Robison JE, Kaye JJ. Simultaneous fractures of the capitate and hamate in the coronal plane: case report. J Hand Surg Am 2005; 30: 1153–1155

Roth JH, de Lorenzi C. Displaced intra-articular coronal fracture of the body of the hamate treated with a Herbert screw. J Hand Surg Am 1988; 13: 619–621

Scheufler O, Radmer S, Erdmann D, Exner K, Germann G, Andresen R. Current treatment of hamate hook fractures. [Article in German.] Handchir Mikrochir Plast Chir 2006; 38: 273–282

Smith P, III, Wright TW, Wallace PF, Dell PC. Excision of the hook of the hamate: a retrospective survey and review of the literature. J Hand Surg Am 1988; 13: 612–615

Walsh JJ, IV, Bishop AT. Diagnosis and management of hamate hook fractures. Hand Clin 2000; 16: 397–403

Intramedullary Kirschner Wire Splinting, Pinning

Blazar PE, Leven D. Intramedullary nail fixation for metacarpal fractures. Hand Clin 2010; 26: 321–325

Cuénod P. Intramedullary fixation of displaced middle phalangeal neck fractures. [Article in French.] Chir Main 2013; 32: 287–291

Dhamangaonkar AC, Patankar HS. Antegrade joint-sparing intramedullary wiring for middle phalanx shaft fractures. J Hand Surg Am 2014; 39: 1517–1523

Foucher G, Chemorin C, Sibilly A. A new technic of osteosynthesis in fractures of the distal 3d of the 5th metacarpus. [Article in French.] Nouv Presse Med 1976; 5: 1139–1140

Foucher G. "Bouquet" osteosynthesis in metacarpal neck fractures: a series of 66 patients. J Hand Surg Am 1995; 20: S86–S90

Förstner H. Intramedullary nailing of distal mid-hand fractures—technique, instruments, case reports. [Article in German.] Handchir Mikrochir Plast Chir 1994; 26: 29–34

Gonzalez MH, Igram CM, Hall RF, Jr. Flexible intramedullary nailing for metacarpal fractures. J Hand Surg Am 1995; 20: 382–387

Gonzalez MH, Igram CM, Hall RF. Intramedullary nailing of proximal phalangeal fractures. J Hand Surg Am 1995; 20: 808–812

Itadera E, Hiwatari R, Moriya H, Ono Y. Closed intramedullary fixation for metacarpal fractures using J-shaped nail. Hand Surg 2008; 13: 139–145

Larkin G, Brüser P, Safi A. Possibilities and limits of intramedullary Kirschner wire osteosynthesis in treatment of metacarpal fractures. [Article in German.] Handchir Mikrochir Plast Chir 1997; 29: 192–196

Mohammed R, Farook MZ, Newman K. Percutaneous elastic intramedullary nailing of metacarpal fractures: surgical technique and clinical results study. J Orthop Surg 2011; 6: 37

Moutet F, Frère G. Metacarpal fractures. [Les fractures des metacarpiens.] Ann Chir Main 1987; 6: 5–14

Orbay JL, Touhami A. The treatment of unstable metacarpal and phalangeal shaft fractures with flexible nonlocking and locking intramedullary nails. Hand Clin 2006; 22: 279–286

Ozer K, Gillani S, Williams A, Peterson SL, Morgan S. Comparison of intramedullary nailing versus plate-screw fixation of extra-articular metacarpal fractures. J Hand Surg Am 2008; 33: 1724–1731

Pelissier P, Recanati G, Alet JM. In-out-in pinning for phalangeal fractures. Chir Main 2015; 34: 24–26

Sandner A, Menke H. Results of antegrade intramedullar Kirschner-Wire pinning of subcapital fracture of the fifth metacarpal bone using Foucher's technique. [Article in German.] Handchir Mikrochir Plast Chir 2008; 40: 336–341

Schädel-Höpfner M, Wild M, Windolf J, Linhart W. Antegrade intramedullary splinting or percutaneous retrograde crossed pinning for displaced neck fractures of the fifth metacarpal? Arch Orthop Trauma Surg 2007; 127: 435–440

Schlageter M, Winkel R, Porcher R, Haas HG. Intramedullary osteosynthesis of distal metacarpal fractures with curved wires. [Article in German.] Handchir Mikrochir Plast Chir 1997; 29: 197–203

Sletten IN, Nordsletten L, Husby T, Ødegaard RA, Hellund JC, Kvernmo HD. Isolated, extra-articular neck and shaft fractures of the 4th and 5th metacarpals: a comparison of transverse and bouquet (intra-medullary) pinning in 67 patients. J Hand Surg Eur Vol 2012; 37: 387–395

Wong TC, Ip FK, Yeung SH. Comparison between percutaneous transverse fixation and intramedullary K-wires in treating closed fractures of the metacarpal neck of the little finger. J Hand Surg [Br] 2006; 31: 61–65

11.9.8 External Fixator

Ashmead D, IV, Rothkopf DM, Walton RL, Jupiter JB. Treatment of hand injuries by external fixation. J Hand Surg Am 1992; 17: 954–964

Dailiana Z, Agorastakis D, Varitimidis S, Bargiotas K, Roidis N, Malizos KN. Use of a mini-external fixator for the treatment of hand fractures. J Hand Surg Am 2009; 34: 630–636

Gausepohl T, Lukosch S, Koebke J, Pennig D. External stabilization of the metacarpal bones II to V. Anatomic-clinical study. [Article in German.] Handchir Mikrochir Plast Chir 1998; 30: 95–102

Houshian S, Jing SS. A new technique for closed management of displaced intra-articular fractures of metacarpal and phalangeal head delayed on presentation: report of eight cases. J Hand Surg Eur Vol 2014; 39: 232–236

Kubitskiy A, Soliman BAB, Dowd MB, Curtin P. External fixation of the hand: a simple approach to comminuted proximal interphalangeal joint fractures. Hand Surg 2014; 19: 85–89

Lenin Babu V, Baskaran K, Kocialkowski A. External fixation of finger fractures made simple. Acta Orthop Belg 2005; 71: 347–348

Mader K, Gausepohl T, Pennig D. Minimally invasive management of metacarpal I fractures with a mini-fixateur. [Article in German.] Handchir Mikrochir Plast Chir 2000; 32: 107–111

Margić K. External fixation of closed metacarpal and phalangeal fractures of digits. A prospective study of one hundred consecutive patients. J Hand Surg [Br] 2006; 31: 30–40

Marsland D, Sanghrajka AP, Goldie B. Static monolateral external fixation for the Rolando fracture: a simple solution for a complex fracture. Ann R Coll Surg Engl 2012; 94: 112–115

Miura T. Extension block pinning using a small external fixator for mallet finger fractures. J Hand Surg Am 2013; 38: 2348–2352

Pennig D, Gausepohl T, Mader K, Wulke A. The use of minimally invasive fixation in fractures of the hand—the minifixator concept. Injury 2000; 31 Suppl 1: 102–112

Schuind F, Noorbergen M, Andrianne Y, Burny F. Comminuted fractures of the base of the first metacarpal treated by distraction-external fixation. J Orthop Trauma 1988; 2: 314–321

Shehadi SI. External fixation of metacarpal and phalangeal fractures. J Hand Surg Am 1991; 16: 544–550

Towfigh H, Theis W. Minifixateur externe zur äußeren Fixation am Handskelett. OP-Journal 1991; 2: 61–67

11.9.9 Adaptive Fixation

Al-Qattan MM. Displaced unstable transverse fractures of the shaft of the proximal phalanx of the fingers in industrial workers: reduction and K-wire fixation leaving the metacarpophalangeal and proximal interphalangeal joints free. J Hand Surg Eur Vol 2011; 36: 577–583

Badia A, Riano F. A simple fixation method for unstable bony mallet finger. J Hand Surg Am 2004; 29: 1051–1055

Belsky MR, Eaton RG, Lane LB. Closed reduction and internal fixation of proximal phalangeal fractures. J Hand Surg Am 1984; 9: 725–729

Damron TA, Engber WD, Lange RH et al. Biomechanical analysis of mallet finger fracture fixation techniques. J Hand Surg Am 1993; 18: 600–607, discussion 608

Eberlin KR, Babushkina A, Neira JR, Mudgal CS. Outcomes of closed reduction and periarticular pinning of base and shaft fractures of the proximal phalanx. J Hand Surg Am 2014; 39: 1524–1528

Egloff C, Sproedt J, Jandali AR. Results after osteosynthesis of extraarticular proximal phalangeal fractures. [Article in German.] Handchir Mikrochir Plast Chir 2012; 44: 5–10

Ender HG, Hintringer W. Die perkutane Versorgung von knöchernen Ausrissen der Strecksehnen und Seitenbänder an den Fingern mit dem "Hakendraht". Unfallchirurgie 1986; 12: 143–147

Faruqui S, Stern PJ, Kiefhaber TR. Percutaneous pinning of fractures in the proximal third of the proximal phalanx: complications and outcomes. J Hand Surg Am 2012; 37: 1342–1348

Franssen BBGM. Kirschner wires: insertion techniques and bone related consequences (Dissertation, Proefschrift). Uni Utrecht; 2010

Freeland AE, Bloom HAT. Percutaneous wiring—principles, techniques, and applications. Curr Orthop 2002; 16: 255–264

Fritz D, Lutz M, Arora R, Gabl M, Wambacher M, Pechlaner S. Delayed single Kirschner wire compression technique for mallet fracture. J Hand Surg [Br] 2005; 30: 180–184

Gehrmann SV, Kaufmann RA, Grassmann JP et al. Fracture-dislocations of the carpometacarpal joints of the ring and little finger. J Hand Surg Eur Vol 2015; 40: 84–87

Greeven AP, Alta TD, Scholtens RE, de Heer P, van der Linden FM. Closed reduction intermetacarpal Kirschner wire fixation in the treatment of unstable fractures of the base of the first metacarpal. Injury 2012; 43: 246–251

Gregory S, Lalonde DH, Fung Leung LT. Minimally invasive finger fracture management: wide-awake closed reduction, K-wire fixation, and early protected movement. Hand Clin 2014; 30: 7–15

Gussous YM, Zhao C, Amadio PC, An KN. The resurgence of barbed suture and connecting devices for use in flexor tendon tenorrhaphy. Hand (NY) 2011; 6: 268–275

Gregory S, Lalonde DH, Fung Leung LT. Minimally invasive finger fracture management: wide-awake closed reduction, K-wire fixation, and early protected movement. Hand Clin 2014; 30: 7–15

Hintringer W, Ender HG. Percutaneous management of intra-articular fractures of the interphalangeal joints of the fingers. [Article in German.] Handchir Mikrochir Plast Chir 18: 356–362

Hoch J, Fritsch H, Frenz C. Are "Busch fracture," "avulsion fracture of the extensor tendon" or "fracture of the dorsal terminal finger joint" synonyms? Anatomic studies of the insertion of the extensor aponeurosis and significance in hand surgery. [Article in German.] Handchir Mikrochir Plast Chir 1994; 26: 237–245

Hofmeister EP, Mazurek MT, Shin AY, Bishop AT. Extension block pinning for large mallet fractures. J Hand Surg Am 2003; 28: 453–459

Horton TC, Hatton M, Davis TR. A prospective randomized controlled study of fixation of long oblique and spiral shaft fractures of the proximal phalanx: closed reduction and percutaneous Kirschner wiring versus open reduction and lag screw fixation. J Hand Surg [Br] 2003; 28: 5–9

Hsu LP, Schwartz EG, Kalainov DM, Chen F, Makowiec RL. Complications of K-wire fixation in procedures involving the hand and wrist. J Hand Surg Am 2011; 36: 610–616

Ishiguro T, Itoh Y, Yabe Y, Hashizume N. Operation des dislozierten knöchernen Strecksehnenausrisses an den Langfingern. Oper Orthop Traumatol 1999; 11: 107–113

Maalla R, Youssef M, Ben Jdidia G, Khimiri C, Essadam H. Extension-block pinning for fracture-dislocation of the proximal interphalangeal joint. Orthop Traumatol Surg Res 2012; 98: 559–563

Matzon JL, Cornwall R. A stepwise algorithm for surgical treatment of type II displaced pediatric phalangeal neck fractures. J Hand Surg Am 2014; 39: 467–473

Nelis R, Wouters DB. Is the use of biodegradable devices in the operative treatment of avulsion fractures of fingers, the so-called mallet finger advantageous? A feasibility study with meniscus arrows. Open Orthop J 2008; 2: 151–154

Olivier LC, Schmidt G, Siemers F, Bong J, Schmit-Neuerburg KP. Lengemann suture versus bone screw osteosynthesis in treatment of ulnar osseous collateral ligament rupture of the thumb metacarpophalangeal joint. [Article in German.] Handchir Mikrochir Plast Chir 1999; 31: 90–95, discussion 96–97

Orhun H, Dursun M, Orhun E, Gürkan V, Altun G. Open reduction and K-wire fixation of mallet finger injuries: mid-term results. [Article in Turkish.] Acta Orthop Traumatol Turc 2009; 43: 395–399

Paksima N, Johnson J, Brown A, Cohn M. Percutaneous pinning of middle phalangeal neck fractures: surgical technique. J Hand Surg Am 2012; 37: 1913–1916

Potenza V, Caterini R, De Maio F, Bisicchia S, Farsetti P. Fractures of the neck of the fifth metacarpal bone. Medium-term results in 28 cases treated by percutaneous transverse pinning. Injury 2012; 43: 242–245

Reck T, Landsleitner B, Richter H, Geldmacher J. A new method of transosseous pull-out wire fixation in ligamentous injuries of the metacarpophalangeal joint of the thumb. [Article in German.] Handchir Mikrochir Plast Chir 1991; 23: 90–92

Reissner L, Gienck M, Weishaupt D, Platz A, Kilgus M. Clinical and radiological results after operative treatment of mallet fracture using Kirschner wire technique. [Article in German.] Handchir Mikrochir Plast Chir 2012; 44: 11–16

Sauerbier M, Krimmer H, Hahn P, Lanz U. Dorsale intraartikuläre Endphalanxfrakturen. Handchir Mikrochir Plast Chir 1999; 31: 82–87, discussion 87–89

Seno N, Hashizume H, Inoue H, Imatani J, Morito Y. Fractures of the base of the middle phalanx of the finger. Classification, management and long-term results. J Bone Joint Surg Br 1997; 79: 758–763

Stern PJ, Kastrup JJ. Complications and prognosis of treatment of mallet finger. J Hand Surg Am 1988; 13: 329–334

Vitale MA, White NJ, Strauch RJ. A percutaneous technique to treat unstable dorsal fracture-dislocations of the proximal interphalangeal joint. J Hand Surg Am 2011; 36: 1453–1459

Waris E, Alanen V. Percutaneous, intramedullary fracture reduction and extension block pinning for dorsal proximal interphalangeal fracture-dislocations. J Hand Surg Am 2010; 35: 2046–2052

Zach A, Lautenbach M, Merk H et al. Frakturen der Phalangen. Handchirurgie Scan 2013;1: 49–65

Zach A. Percutaneous fixation of transverse shaft fractures of the proximal phalanx with a new compression wire. J Hand Surg Eur Vol 2015; 40: 318–319

Zhang X, Shao X, Huang Y. Pullout wire fixation together with distal interphalangeal joint Kirschner wire stabilization for acute combined tendon and bone (double level) mallet finger injury. J Hand Surg Am 2015; 40: 363–367

11.9.10 Dynamic Distraction External Fixation

Badia A, Riano F, Ravikoff J, Khouri R, Gonzalez-Hernandez E, Orbay JL. Dynamic intradigital external fixation for proximal interphalangeal joint fracture dislocations. J Hand Surg Am 2005; 30: 154–160

Bayer-Sandow T, Brüser P. The dynamic treatment of intraarticular fractures of the base of the middle phalanx with the Suzuki dynamic fixator. [Article in German.] Handchir Mikrochir Plast Chir 2001; 33: 267–270

Damert H-G, Altmann S, Kraus A, Infanger M, Sattler D. Treatment of intraarticular middle phalanx fractures using the Ligamentotaxor®. Hand (NY) 2013; 8: 460–463

Duteille F, Pasquier P, Lim A, Dautel G. Treatment of complex interphalangeal joint fractures with dynamic external traction: a series of 20 cases. Plast Reconstr Surg 2003; 111: 1623–1629

Ellis SJ, Cheng R, Prokopis P et al. Treatment of proximal interphalangeal dorsal fracture-dislocation injuries with dynamic external fixation: a pins and rubber band system. J Hand Surg Am 2007; 32: 1242–1250

Goldberg E, Unglaub F, Kneser U, Horch RE. Intraarticular fractures of the proximal interphalangeal joint: dynamic early functional therapy with an external fixation system. [Article in German.] Unfallchirurg 2009; 112: 337–345

Henn CM, Lee SK, Wolfe SW. Dynamic external fixation for proximal interphalangeal fracture-dislocations. Oper Tech Orthop 2012; 22: 142–150

Kiral A, Erken HY, Akmaz I, Yildirim C, Erler K. Pins and rubber band traction for treatment of comminuted intra-articular fractures in the hand. J Hand Surg Am 2014; 39: 696–705

Körting O, Facca S, Diaconu M, Liverneaux P. Treatment of complex proximal interphalangeal joint fractures using a new dynamic external fixator: 15 cases. Chir Main 2009; 28: 153–157

Lee JYL, Teoh LC. Dorsal fracture dislocations of the proximal interphalangeal joint treated by open reduction and interfragmentary screw fixation: indications, approaches and results. J Hand Surg [Br] 2006; 31: 138–146

Mansha M, Miranda S. Early results of a simple distraction dynamic external fixator in management of comminuted intra-articular fractures of base of middle phalanx. J Hand Microsurg 2013; 5: 63–67

Richter M, Brüser P. Long term follow-up of fracture dislocations and comminuted fractures of the PIP joint treated with Suzuki's pin and rubber traction system. [Article in German.] Handchir Mikrochir Plast Chir 2008; 40: 330–335

Ruland RT, Hogan CJ, Cannon DL, Slade JF. Use of dynamic distraction external fixation for unstable fracture-dislocations of the proximal interphalangeal joint. J Hand Surg Am 2008; 33: 19–25

Suzuki Y, Matsunaga T, Sato S, Yokoi T. The pins and rubbers traction system for treatment of comminuted intraarticular fractures and fracture-dislocations in the hand. J Hand Surg [Br] 1994; 19: 98–107

11.9.11 Hook Plate

Cheah AEJ, Tan DM, Chong AK, Chew WY. Volar plating for unstable proximal interphalangeal joint dorsal fracture-dislocations. J Hand Surg Am 2012; 37: 28–33

Szalay G, Schleicher I, Kraus R, Pavlidis T, Schnettler R. Operative treatment of the mallet fracture using a hook plate. [Article in German.] Handchir Mikrochir Plast Chir 2011; 43: 46–53

Teoh LC, Lee JY. Mallet fractures: a novel approach to internal fixation using a hook plate. J Hand Surg Eur Vol 2007; 32: 24–30

11.9.12 Absorbable Pins

Haas HG. PDS splint in the treatment of fractures. [Article in German.] Handchir Mikrochir Plast Chir 1986; 18: 295–297

Gunatillake PA, Adhikari R. Biodegradable synthetic polymers for tissue engineering. Eur Cell Mater 2003; 5: 1–16, discussion 16

Rustemeier M, Ganssmann M. Treatment of osseous ruptures of the flexor tendons with resorbable materials. [Article in German.] Handchir Mikrochir Plast Chir 1986; 18: 302–303

Wüstner MC, Partecke BD, Buck-Gramcko D. Resorbable PDS splints in fracture stabilization and for arthrodeses of the hand. [Article in German.] Handchir Mikrochir Plast Chir 1986; 18: 298–301

Index